NOT FALLING

Fall Prevention Strategies

A Roadmap for Patients and Caregivers

MARTIN MENKIN, M.D.

ISBN: 978-1-7369303-0-4

Cover design: David James

Printed in the United States of America

CONTENTS

INTRODUCTION

Men occasionally stumble over the truth, but most of them pick themselves up and hurry off as if nothing had happened.

— Winston Churchill

According to the theory of evolution, the ancient ancestors of man lived as lower life forms drifting at the whim of the sea, in a planetary amniotic space. Random changes confronted the circumstances of life. Adaptations that offered benefit were selected to persist. Bipedal gait was selected, and this mode of locomotion became obligatory as man was challenged to transition from living in the trees to dwelling on the ground. Obligate bipedal gait carries an unrelenting risk of falling. The responsibility for not falling rests on man alone.

One in three Americans over 65 years of age fell last year.[1] One every two seconds. 16 million people. That's greater than the combined populations of New York, Los Angeles, Chicago, and Houston each year. Over 1.5 million of these people required care in an emergency room. Some required admission to the hospital for an average stay of 7.9 days, with an average cost of $35,000.[2] Over 20,000 people died as a consequence of their fall. Cruel? Perhaps. But perhaps not hopeless. Falling may not be inevitable if we formulate a proper plan!

The direct cost of falls each year in the United States is $50 billion. This is estimated to rise to $240 billion by the year 2040.[3] Additional indirect costs to caregiver families in the form of time, effort, and lost productivity are difficult to quantify, but are substantial. Even an expensive plan to reduce falls might actually save money.

United States governmental agencies such as the National Institute of Health (NIH), Center for Disease Control (CDC), Housing and Urban Development (HUD), and others spend millions of dollars each year on programs to inform the public, teach healthcare providers, perform research, and administer research grants at academic centers. Many more millions are spent by public service organizations, health insurance companies, not-for-profit foundations and for-profit corporations. Extensive research is done by the governments of other countries and international agencies such as the World Health Organization. It is money well spent.

Thousands of meaningful studies and recommendations are generated each year. Studies are published in magazines and in scientific journals, and online. A simple internet search on "fall prevention" will turn up thousands of articles, research studies, YouTube presentations, and blogs. Informative pamphlets are distributed at doctors' offices and emergency rooms. It is strikingly easy to find accurate and thorough information on the subject. And yet, people continue to fall. We need a better plan. We need to plan better.

A proper plan has an anatomy. It begins with the recognition of a starting point followed by a stated purpose and/or anticipated goal. In a plan for fall prevention, that starting point is intentional upright bipedal gait, and the goal is to reduce pain and increase productivity by reducing the number and severity of falls. A plan must have, as its core, a path that actually achieves this goal. The combination of purpose and path is properly called *a strategy*.

A strategy, even a good one, might work or it might fail. It requires courage to pursue a strategy in the face of this uncertainty. But courage is not a strategy. Courage untethered to wisdom can be foolish. You don't want to spend a lot of time and money on "foolish." There should be some reasonable hope that a wise plan, executed with courage, will achieve the goal. But hope is also not a strategy. Hope is a lens through which you can perceive the benefits of courage in the face of uncertainty.

Tactics are tools which, when executed with hope and courage, achieve an objective. The purpose and path of a strategy pursue the cumulative consequences of carefully chosen tactics. Addressing several different objectives may be necessary to achieve a goal. As a specific example, in a plan to reduce the risk for recurrent falls, the objectives of the tactics are divided into two domains: objectives which are extrinsic to the person and objectives which are intrinsic to the person. Each domain requires a different set of tactics.

A working understanding of the difference between the intrinsic and the extrinsic causes of falling is of critical importance. Tactics must be selected to address objectives, both intrinsic and extrinsic, or the strategic plan will be an incomplete success. Rehabilitation of defective balance mechanisms does not effectively reduce falls related to environmental hazards. The extensive work already done in the field of fall prevention as well as future efforts must be viewed from this perspective.

Despite this lack of strategic clarity, vast work has been done in the field of fall prevention. Much of it is intelligent, accurate, and enlightening, while a small portion is misleading, contradictory, or methodologically flawed.

New thinking reveals new conjectures on a daily basis. For the researcher, and the computer-skilled persistent elderly, computers offer efficient access to a tremendous volume of literature. A useful partial list of internet resources is included in Appendix A. But many people have limited access to the Internet, especially the elderly, and many others might wish to visit the subject without the constant distractions of digital links. For those who value circumscribed thinking and a consistent perspective, this book will be a more accessible and useful alternative.

This book offers a perspective on the strategy and tactics to reduce falling for everyone, especially elderly adults. If this simply recasts the work of others in a new light, it will be an accessible supplement to the many excellent sources on the topic of falls prevention.

Chapter 1 brings the extrinsic factors for falling into clear focus, and in doing so, existing strategies are refocused. Chapter 2 redefines the role of intrinsic factors for falling, and to some extent, breaks new ground. Chapter 3 reviews new and innovative options which are just now becoming available, or have been available and are just now being applied. These are thoughts about what can occur in the near future to reduce falls and rehabilitate individuals with gait/balance disorders.

This book is written primarily for those who have fallen and for their caregivers. It is also for those who recognize that they are at risk for falling in the future and would like to do something to avoid the pain, cost, and loss of independence. Additionally, it will be a resource for physicians caring for patients at risk, and a guidepost to policymakers and stakeholders working in their communities.

One speculation in Chapter 3, a section on "adaptation by regressive genetic expression," clearly lacks scientific proof. Such is the nature of speculation. If by including this, I "am hoist on my own petard," my critics are referred to what "Doc Jess" Meredith from Fancy Gap, Virginia told me in 1968. He memorably assured this Yankee medical student in an orientation lecture on how to speak proper *Southern*: "Even a blind pig finds an acorn sometimes."

NOTES

[1] Overcoming Obstacles to Effective Senior Falls Prevention and Coordinated Care, https://www.hud.gov/sites/documents/SENIORFALLS_TOOLKIT.PDF.

[2] "Medical Costs of Fatal and Nonfatal Falls in Older Adults," Curtis S. Florence, PhD,* Gwen Bergen, PhD,* Adam Atherly, PhD, †Elizabeth Burns, MPH,*Judy Stevens, PhD,* and Cynthia Drake, MA†, *Journal of the American Geriatric Society,* April 2018 66: 693-698 https://doi.org/10.1111/jgs.15304.

[3] The Cost of Fall Injuries Among Older Adults, https://nfsi.org/wp-content/uploads/2013/10/Costs.pdf.

CHAPTER 1
EXTRINSIC FACTORS

We are continually faced by great opportunities brilliantly disguised as insoluble problems.

— Lee Iacocca

The majority of elderly adults say that they wish to never move from their home. Over time, the place has become familiar and predictable. It is the neighborhood — "home is where you can walk to." It is the vessel for memories that grow more cherished with each passing decade. But with aging comes limitations. The house and the yard and the neighborhood that were so accommodating at age 50, are no longer fully satisfactory for an 80-year-old. The once nurturing environment has become hazardous.

Surroundings have character. They can be bright or dark, or roiled by contrasting light. They may take on human attributes. Quiet can be soothing, indifferent, or spooky. A spacious room with good natural light is accommodating and friendly. A well-placed grab-bar is firm and assuring. Factors that favor risk or harm are hostile — even demonic. A hazardous dark stairway is threatening and frightful. "Hazard" is from the Arabic "Az-zahr" — a game of dice. Uncertain. Risky. Dicey. Not invariably harmful, but with the potential for harm. Random risk on the one hand, potentially avoidable on the other. Lucifer fell from heaven and gave us hazards. As Shakespeare's King Lear admonishes his daughter to ""mend your speech a little, lest it mar your fortune," so extrinsic hazards say, "mend your environment a little, lest it mar your health."

Extrinsic risks for falling permeate the environment. They are the cumulative consequence of two categories. The most easily envisioned are universally experienced environmental circumstances such as wet floors, poor lighting, holes in the walkway, and such. The extrinsic risks that are less easily identified arise from the extrinsic influences of socio-demographic factors. This refers to extrinsic risks for which exposure might be limited to, for example, the poor, health-care workers, and retirees. How to reduce extrinsic risks is a fertile area for analysis, innovation, and education.

The most reasonable solution is to identify the hazard and remove it. There is a small body of research that suggests that the problem lies with people, not things. It suggests that the identification and elimination of environmental hazards offers little or no benefit in the home setting. But an overwhelming majority of research studies indicate that management of extrinsic risks for falling reduces falls in the home by anywhere from 30% to as much as 80%. The lack of uniform agreement among research studies is due, in large part, to the lack of uniformity in how the studies are conducted. This is unavoidable. It results from the high number of environmental and individual variables that must be taken into account. In part, it is because hazards are not uniformly distributed among socio-demographic groups. Hopefully, ongoing research will lend more clarity. In the meantime, the elderly, caregivers, policy makers, and public and private agencies should continue to work to reduce hazards. This has been proven to reduce falls in the workplace[4] and almost certainly works to reduce falls at home.

SECTION 1
Hazard Modification: The Built Environment

The most evident extrinsic risks for falling arise from hazards encountered connected to the structural aspects of the environment. This a subset of the general environment referred to as "the built environment." This refers to those things, manufactured and built, with which we interact on a daily basis.

Hazards in the built environment exist in two domains. Some lie within the home and others exist outside of the home, in the yard or in the community. Each domain harbors unique risk factors to which unique tactics apply. Those risks for falling in the home and immediately outside of the home, in the yard are often reduced by thoughtful observation and intuitive corrective measures. Those in the community often require policy and funding that prioritize fall prevention over other community needs. The elements of weather, rain, ice and snow, are aspects of extrinsic risk that occur in the community and in the yard. Mud, ice, and standing water cannot be neglected either. The environmental factors of global warming and pollution will probably soon be included as well. Someday, populations at risk will suffer more falls when coastal fisheries produce less food or at the time of some alternate ecosystem collapse. For now, vast islands of floating plastic in the Pacific Ocean will not make a person fall. But a single plastic bottle lurking on the third stair might be lethal today to anyone, anywhere.

Fall risk reduction in the built environment can be approached in two ways. Both approaches focus on *Hazard Modification*. The first involves identifying and eliminating existing hazards. This approach, based on observation and intuition, has years of proven success. It is accomplished by performing a thoughtful audit of the home or community environment using a checklist. The identified hazard is then removed or corrected. The second approach to reducing the risk of falls is to redesign the built environment to fit the needs of all people, young, old, able-bodied, and otherwise. This is based on principles of architecture and social science, first initiated 50 years ago, which seem to show clear benefit in recent years. It is referred to as modification based on Universal Design. This approach is to build (or rebuild) with the goal to allow universal use — that is, a home or a yard or a town that can be accessed fully and used safely by anyone. It is a key component to a behavioral goal referred to as "Aging in Place."

Observation and intuition are the earliest tools that brought meaningful benefit in reducing existing hazards. Recommendations based on observation and intuition work, and with more systematic review in recent years, our tactics have been refined. The main tactic is a proper checklist.

SECTION 2
Hazard Modification: Checklists

Good checklists...are precise. They do not spell out everything. Instead, they provide reminders of the most critical and important steps...the ones that even the highly skilled professional using them could miss. Good checklists are, above all, practical.

— Atul Gawande, *Being Mortal*

An essay is a discourse on a subject — a complete thought. It is often written in order to define a circumstance, and then suggest a response to that circumstance. At its best, an essay can reveal order where there is the appearance of chaos, and can focus attention where there has been indifference. A checklist can do the same thing. It can do it better than an essay if the complete thought entails multiple circumstances. This is especially true when the multiple circumstances that are being addressed distribute logically in "clusters." An essay on what is missing from the pantry is not as useful as a grocery list. And, a grocery checklist works best when fruits and vegetables are clustered together. A checklist list is more than an essay for the dyslexic. It is a tool. It needs to be a good one.

The tactic is to use this checklist tool. The task is to get people to employ the tactic. No benefit is realized until a person with need performs the checklist-driven audit of their home and then follows the recommendation to remove the hazard. This task is easier when the checklist makes sense. Even indifferent and skeptical people can embrace common sense. A good checklist addresses circumstances in an orderly, rational, and practical fashion. The checklist format risks being neglected if it meanders indifferently between locations or includes nonsense. It must engender trust. Regrettably, even a stunning checklist might not inspire the desired behavior. Some tactics are best done by a third party on behalf of the person with need.

In addition to being trustworthy, a checklist has other virtues. A checklist consists of thoughts masquerading as tasks. It is something that even a procrastinator might eventually begin. The task can be stopped and restarted, or even partially ignored, and still offer some benefit. It is impersonal. It can be a "third party" instrument, proctored by a total stranger. This may actually be viewed by some elderly as less intrusive than a survey done by a relative. It is both objective and thorough.

A checklist for extrinsic fall risks has no mandatory format. The most logical checklists have clusters of tasks based on the location of the risk. The checklist for a particular location, such as the kitchen, lists risk circumstances that exist at that location. It then offers an appropriate recommendation, or a list of recommendations, designed to modify that risk. Each location checklist should stand alone.

A different checklist is created for each location, but there is redundancy. The risk "loose carpet" will appear in the checklist as a circumstance of concern for each location at which loose carpets might occur such as on stairs, in a hallway, or in a living room. This circumstance is then followed by a recommendation to tack down the loose edge. Some recommendations will, therefore, be repeated for several locations in a redundant fashion. Others, like "place a light switch at both the top and bottom of the stairway" will be available only in the checklist for stairs.

The risk circumstance and the recommendation will each have a box for a checkmark. Later, when the survey of the home and yard is completed, the checkmarks are reviewed, or audited, to provide a "to do" list of recommended measures. The inclusion of an "Anywhere" location can list generalized afterthoughts, such as "always be alert and careful." This is perhaps best preceded by a statement such as "generalized afterthoughts are a regrettable necessity."

State and local governments, public interest groups, private not-for-profit organizations, private companies, church-based support groups, and multiple federal agencies (to name a few) have published pamphlets with checklists designed to reduce falls. All are similar. Each is useful. None are perfect. What follows is a reasonable effort to combine the efforts of others[5, 6, 7, 8] in the empathetic, if vain, hope that combining three or four very good lists will yield a single best list.

Home Hazard Modification Checklist

STAIRS

- ☐ Clutter on stairwell or landings in the form of boxes, books, clothes, shoes, other objects?

  - ☐ Remove the clutter.

  - ☐ Avoid return of clutter in coming months.

- ☐ Electrical wires or a phone cable on the landing or in the stairwell?

  - ☐ Remove wires and cables.

  - ☐ Firmly secure wires or cables out of way along the wall.

- ☐ Furniture blocks walkway at top or bottom of stairs?

  - ☐ Move the furniture to permit safe passage.

  - ☐ Remove furniture from the area at the top or bottom of stairs.

- ☐ Carpet is present with unsecured edges or an irregular surface?

  - ☐ Tack down the edges of the carpet.

  - ☐ Remove or replace worn-out carpet.

- ☐ Lighting insufficient or difficult to use?

  - ☐ Install light switches at top and bottom of stairs. Consider motion-sensing switches.

  - ☐ Install ceiling fixtures that light the entire stairway.

  - ☐ Install nightlights. Consider a motion-sensing type.

☐ Reduce excess glare from lighting with proper light bulb selection.

☐ Reduce excess glare with proper ceiling fixture selection.

☐ Consider placing visible tape or paint on the front edge of each stair and landing.

☐ Handrails are missing, loose, or in disrepair?

    ☐ Add handrails to both sides of stairwell.

    ☐ Repair or replace an loose or broken handrails by anchoring to framing.

☐ Stairs are broken, loose, or otherwise in disrepair?

    ☐ Repair or replace the treads (the part you step on).

    ☐ Repair or replace the risers (the vertical board at the front edge of the tread).

☐ Stairs are slick or slippery?

    ☐ Apply non-skid surface in the form of tack-down strips, runners, tape, or paint designed for this purpose.

☐ One stair or two stair step-downs are located anywhere in the house?

    ☐ Mark these with visible tape or paint to make them more visible.

HALLWAY

☐ Clutter on the floor in the form of boxes, books, clothes, shoes, other objects?

  ☐ Remove the clutter

  ☐ Avoid return of clutter in coming months.

☐ Electrical wires and phone cable present in the area?

  ☐ Remove wires and cables.

  ☐ Firmly secure wires and cables out of the way along the wall.

☐ Furniture blocks hallway?

  ☐ Move furniture to permit safe passage.

  ☐ Remove the furniture from the area.

☐ Thresholds and doorsills elevated?

  ☐ Lower doorsills and thresholds as much as possible.

  ☐ Mark thresholds and doorsills with tape or paint for visibility.

☐ Carpet with unsecured edges or irregular surface?

  ☐ Tack down edges of carpet or secure with two-sided carpet tape.

  ☐ Remove unsecured throw rugs.

☐ Lighting poor or difficult to use?

  ☐ Install nightlights.

- ☐ Maintain easy access to light switches by moving furniture and/or relocating switches.

- ☐ Install light switches at both ends of hallway.

- ☐ Add ceiling fixtures as needed.

- ☐ Adjust fixtures and bulbs to avoid excess glare from lighting.

☐ Floor is slippery or slick?

- ☐ use non-skid floor surfaces such as unpolished wood or low, dense pile carpet

BEDROOM

☐ Clutter on the floor in the form of boxes, books, clothes, shoes, other objects?

- ☐ Remove the clutter.

- ☐ Remove clutter on the pathway to the bathroom

- ☐ Remove clutter on floor and other areas of closets.

☐ Electrical wires and/or phone cable are in the area?

- ☐ Remove wires and cable.

- ☐ Firmly secure wires and cables out of the way along the wall.

☐ Furniture blocking anticipated walkways, including the pathway to the bathroom?

- ☐ Move furniture to permit safe passage

- ☐ Remove the blocking furniture from the area entirely.

- [ ] Give special attention to furniture blocking the pathway to the bathroom

- [ ] Thresholds and doorsills elevated?

  - [ ] Lower doorsills and thresholds as much as possible.

  - [ ] Mark doorsills with tape or paint for visibility.

- [ ] Carpet present with unsecured edges or irregular surface?

  - [ ] Tack down edges of carpet or secure with two-sided tape.

  - [ ] Remove unsecured throw rugs.

  - [ ] Change carpets to low, dense pile with a simple pattern that is not distracting.

- [ ] Lighting insufficient or difficult to use?

  - [ ] Install a light switch that is easily reached near the bedroom door.

  - [ ] Install nightlights. Consider light/dark sensor and movement sensor-equipped nightlights.

  - [ ] Add lamp at bedside, with a switch at the base of the lamp.

  - [ ] Give special attention to clearly lighting the pathway to and from the bathroom

  - [ ] Reduce excess glare from lighting with use of lamp shades.

  - [ ] Reduce excess glare with use of window treatments.

- [ ] Furniture height, shape, or stability increases the risk of falling when getting up and down?

☐ Change furniture which is too low that may not permit easy standing or transfers.

☐ Add furniture with stable arm supports to assist in getting up.

☐ Remove furniture which is too unsteady or flimsy to support someone leaning on it

☐ Bed is too low? (The correct height supports the upper leg at a horizontal position when the person is seated on the edge of the bed.)

☐ Phone and flashlight access not ideal?

   ☐ Place a phone at the bedside.

   ☐ Consider adding a phone at floor level in case someone has fallen and cannot get up.

   ☐ Place a flashlight at the bedside.

   ☐ Place a wireless doorbell system at the bedside in order to summon assistance from within the home if necessary.

☐ Bathroom pathway is difficult or unsafe to negotiate?

   ☐ Remove clutter along the pathway.

   ☐ Move any furniture obstructing the pathway.

   ☐ Give special attention to lighting of the pathway.

   ☐ Change to an alternate bedroom to permit better access to a bathroom.

   ☐ Make a bedside commode available for night-time use.

BATHROOM

- ☐ Clutter on the floor in the form of garbage pail, towels, clothes, shoes, other objects?

  - ☐ Remove the clutter.

  - ☐ Avoid return of clutter in coming months.

- ☐ Electrical wires present in the area?

  - ☐ Remove wires from the area.

  - ☐ Firmly secure wires that are on countertop areas.

- ☐ Furniture blocking the entry to the bathroom or pathway to the sink, shower, or toilet?

  - ☐ Move the furniture to permit unobstructed passage.

  - ☐ Remove the furniture from the area.

- ☐ Thresholds and doorsills elevated?

  - ☐ Lower doorsills and thresholds as much as possible.

  - ☐ Mark thresholds with bright reflective tape or paint to improve visibility.

- ☐ Lighting poor or difficult to use?

  - ☐ Maintain easy access to light switches or relocate them.

  - ☐ Add ceiling fixtures as needed.

  - ☐ Install nightlights.

  - ☐ Reduce excess glare from lighting by changing light bulbs.

  - ☐ Reduce excess glare with window treatments.

☐ Grab bars for reliable and secure hand holds absent?

   ☐ Replace or remove towel bars. They might appear to be secure, *but are not.*

   ☐ Install horizontal or vertical grab bars, anchoring them solidly into the wall framing.

   ☐ Locate one bar within reach of the toilet.

   ☐ Locate one or two bars on the inside of the shower or bathtub.

   ☐ Locate one bars on the outside of the shower or bathtub.

☐ Bathtub or shower areas slick or slippery, especially when wet?

   ☐ Place rubber bathmats and non-slip strips or silicon decals on the floor of the bathtub or shower

   ☐ Use non-skid bathmats for areas outside the bathtub or shower as well as for other wet areas.

   ☐ Make a bathtub seat or shower bench available for easy use — and encourage their use.

   ☐ Install an adjustable shower head.

   ☐ Install non-skid tiles to the extent possible in the shower and the remainder of the bath area.

   ☐ Create a convenient system to dry wet areas immediately, such a mop or Swifter.

   ☐ Replace bar soap and shampoo bottles with dispensers for those in order to avoid spills.

☐ The toilet has not been changed in any way to reduce falls?

   ☐ Install an elevated toilet seat or commode chair.

   ☐ Install adjustable-height toilet safety frame (toilet safety rails).

   ☐ Facilitate ability to get up from the toilet with a grab bar and/or commode chair arms.

   ☐ Make toilet paper easy to reach, without leaning off-balance.

☐ Shelves are cluttered or disorganized?

   ☐ Organize counters and shelves to make regularly used items easy to reach

KITCHEN

☐ Clutter in the form of boxes, papers, rarely used small appliances, pots, or other objects?

   ☐ Remove the clutter from the floor

   ☐ Avoid the return of clutter in coming months.

   ☐ Remove or organize the clutter on countertops.

   ☐ Remove the clutter from commonly used shelves, cabinets, and drawers.

☐ Electrical wires and phone cable present in the area?

   ☐ Remove wires and cables.

- ☐ Firmly secure wires or cables in an out of the way area along the wall

☐ Furniture blocking commonly used walkways?

- ☐ Move furniture to a location that permits getting around it safely.
- ☐ Remove furniture from the area.

☐ Thresholds and doorsills elevated?

- ☐ Lower doorsills and thresholds as much as possible.
- ☐ Mark doorsills with tape or paint for visibility.

☐ Carpet present with unsecured edges or irregular surface?

- ☐ Tack down edges of carpet or secure with two-sided tape.
- ☐ Remove unsecured throw rugs.

☐ Lighting is insufficient, or difficult to use, or adds too much glare?

- ☐ Maintain easy access to light switches by moving small appliances.
- ☐ Add light switches at each door entering the room. Consider motion-sensing switches.
- ☐ Add ceiling fixtures.
- ☐ Add task lighting.
- ☐ Reduce excess glare from lighting by changing light bulbs.

- ☐ Reduce excess glare by changing ceiling fixtures, adding dimmer switches, and/or adding window curtains.

- ☐ Install motion-sensing nightlights.

- ☐ Pots, dishes and other commonly used items on shelves and in cabinets which are difficult to access?

  - ☐ Move commonly used kitchen items to lower shelves to avoid needing to reach or climb.

  - ☐ Move commonly used kitchen items out of low, deep cabinets to avoid needing to bend down.

  - ☐ Avoid step stools. If really needed, get one that is ideally stable with an upper handrail.

  - ☐ Place a reaching-stick grabber in convenient location in kitchen.

- ☐ Furniture stability and shape introduces difficulty getting up and down safely?

  - ☐ Replace any unsteady chairs or stools.

  - ☐ Add chairs with firm armrests to assist in standing up.

- ☐ Slippery areas might occur from spilled water or other liquids?

  - ☐ Create a system for wiping up water or spilled liquids immediately.

  - ☐ Avoid use of wax on floors.

  - ☐ Replace flooring with textured tile, laminate, or vinyl that is less likely to become slick.

LIVING ROOM

- ☐ Clutter on the floor and commonly used areas such as boxes, books, clothes, shoes, or other objects?

  - ☐ Remove any clutter on the floor.

  - ☐ Reduce clutter in commonly used cabinets and countertop areas.

- ☐ Electrical wires and phone cable present in the area?

  - ☐ Remove wires and cables.

  - ☐ Firmly secure wires or cables out of the way along the wall.

- ☐ Furniture blocking the frequently used walkways?

  - ☐ Move furniture to permit safe, unobstructed movement.

  - ☐ Remove unnecessary furniture from the area.

- ☐ Thresholds and doorsills elevated?

  - ☐ Lower doorsills and thresholds as much as possible.

  - ☐ Mark thresholds and doorsills with bright reflective tape or paint for visibility.

- ☐ Carpet present with unsecured edges or irregular surface?

  - ☐ Tack down edges of carpet or secure with two-sided tape.

  - ☐ Remove unsecured throw rugs.

- ☐ Lighting is poor or difficult to use?

  - ☐ Install motion-sensing or other nightlights.

☐ Maintain easy access to light switches by moving furniture or relocating switches.

☐ Add lamps and ceiling fixtures as needed.

☐ Reduce excess glare from lighting with lamp shades.

☐ Reduce excess glare with curtains or other window treatments.

☐ Furniture height, shape, or stability makes getting up and down safely difficult?

 ☐ Change furniture that is too low to permit easy and safe transfers.

 ☐ Add furniture with stable arm supports to assist in getting up.

 ☐ Remove unsteady or flimsy furniture that cannot be leaned on safely.

 ☐ Remove furniture that is low or out of sight which might trip someone.

OUTSIDE THE HOUSE

☐ Clutter on the grounds and sidewalks in the form of garbage cans, rocks, plant debris, or other objects?

 ☐ Dispose of the clutter.

 ☐ Avoid return of clutter in coming months.

 ☐ Move objects that are to be kept away from walkways and stairs.

- ☐ Clear driveway, sidewalks, and stairs of roots, branches, and plant debris.

☐ Sidewalks or driveway uneven?

- ☐ Remove elevated edges in a sidewalk by cutting the concrete slab with a concrete saw.

- ☐ Even up edges in a sidewalk by adding concrete to a low slab or by having it lifted from below with polyurethane injection.

- ☐ Fill holes in cement and slate sidewalks, and in dirt pathways.

- ☐ Reset raised bricks and otherwise smooth out brick and cobblestone walkways.

- ☐ Fill holes and repair uneven areas in driveways.

- ☐ Fill holes and remove large rocks from the area immediately beside sidewalks.

- ☐ Fill holes in gardens and garden pathways and remove rocks that can be trip hazards.

☐ Stairs uneven or without rails?

- ☐ Install suitable outdoor stair rails on both sides.

- ☐ Repair broken or uneven steps.

☐ Lighting insufficient in driveway, walkway, stairs, or doorway?

- ☐ Install entrance area lighting.

- ☐ Install sidewalk and driveway lighting.

ANYWHERE

Perhaps this heading should be "everywhere." It does not match the clustered-by-location checklist. What follows fits more into the idea that "generalized afterthoughts are a regrettable necessity."

☐ Do you know the behaviors that can increase the risk of falling in the home?

☐ Carry less. Carry only the amount that you can do so safely.

☐ Carry things in one hand on stairs so that the other hand is free to grasp the handrail.

☐ Carry packages or large objects such that your vision isn't blocked.

☐ Stand up slowly and with caution to reduce dizziness and/or light-headed moments.

☐ Answer the phone or the doorbell without rushing.

☐ Use the commode seated and get up slowly and carefully.

☐ Wear shoes which are supportive and fit well. Avoid floppy slippers, flip-flops, and raised heels, but also avoid walking around barefoot.

☐ Keep track of pets that might get underfoot in the home or during walks.

☐ Wipe up spills immediately and avoid walking in wet areas.

☐ Pay attention. Be careful. Be alert. Don't be distracted

SECTION 3
Hazard Modification: Sociodemographic Risk

The second approach to extrinsic risks recognizes the reality that not all people face the same types of hazards. Social and/or demographic factors can create environments which expose some individuals to unique risk circumstances. For example, a person with low income interacts with environmental hazards differently than someone of higher income.

Anyone can fall in a poorly lit stairwell. Poor lighting is more common in a rental tenement than in a Park Avenue apartment. Insufficient lighting will be readily addressed by a financially secure owner, but is likely to be neglected by an owner with more limited financial resources. A tenant can ask for better lighting, but he might not do so for fear he will be invited to move if he asks for too much. Falls can occur after tripping on a raised sidewalk, but a Caucasian female from a northern state carries a greater risk of hip fracture because of her higher degree of osteoporosis. A woman is more likely to fall inside the home than a man due to a differential incidence of bladder urgency and incontinence. In the yard, a man is more likely to fall than a woman due to the differential incidence of risk behaviors like climbing and digging. Obese people are 31% more likely to fall and 50% less likely to think they can do anything about it.[9] A rutted pathway to the barn does not exist in a metropolitan area. Reducing the hazard remains the tool that needs to be utilized. The tactics to apply the tool must take into account these differential risks.

Section 4
Home Modification: Staying Home

The tactic of observation and intuition works best on binary questions — simple issues that might be called "low hanging fruit." This is the wheelhouse of checklists. Is the tile outside the shower wet? Yes or no? But floors are not simply wet or dry. They also have textures and sheen, and variations of compliance.

Falls clearly occur on poorly lighted stairs, but they can also increase on stairs that are too brightly lighted as well. Intuition does not predict that.

What is the safest height for a countertop? That depends. Is the user in a wheelchair? And, it should also be noted that intuition will never be an acceptable way to deal with the sensitive and nuanced factors of socio-demographic risk.

A checklist proves insufficient in a world with complex questions and multiple options. In order to find answers to the harder non-binary questions we must look to science for evidence-based answers that use data analysis to distinguish between facts and wishes. For example, architectural and social science advances are now being applied to the complex questions of how and where to live as we age. The hope is to gain answers that reduce falls. Current studies demonstrate that this hope is reasonable.[10]

Architecture brings the promise of success in fall prevention and safety in general with a concept called "Universal Design." This term refers to the design and composition of a home (or city environment) in which safe and user-friendly access is assured to all people to the greatest extent possible.

Think about form and function. Early huts and shacks took a form that was a consequence of the anticipated function. Shelter was created. Warmth was retained. Cooking and eating found a place indoors. But over the centuries, form drifted. Large homes took on forms that neglected function in favor of stylish whims. The design of a home grew to favor the artistic preferences of the architect, the uninformed egocentric wishes of the owner, and the pragmatic limitations of the builder.

In the United States, a house built for an average young family during the last 75 years will probably have features that make it a risky place for a older senior adult to live, or for a disabled friend to visit. For example, there may be poor bathroom access or second-story bedrooms.

Recently, there has been a growing awareness of a new option. A home with Universal Design accommodates a visit by anyone (*visitability*), including, for example, a visit by someone in a wheelchair even though no one living there is wheelchair dependent. It turns egocentric whimsical design back toward design where form follows function, and the functions include those of people with limitations or disabilities. — real people.

Whether in the kitchen or bathroom or in the community, Universal Design works to anticipate and accommodate the broad range of human functional capacity, including the limited capacities of advanced-age adults. When thoughtfully done, this can be accomplished without causing the home to look like a rehabilitation clinic, and it can actually increase the resale value of a home. Home modifications are primarily designed for visitability and safety. Research confirms that this hospitable form-follows-function design results in fewer falls.[11]

The "to-do" list identified on a home audit checklist could be considered modifications. Many of the things on this list are simple tasks that you or a family member can do at little cost, such as moving furniture to establish a clear pathway to the bathroom. Some tasks require more.

Setting the hot water maximum temperature to 120 degrees should not be done incorrectly, and simple flooring issues, or installing a raised toilet seat, may require a trip to the store and the use of some simple tools. Large jobs may require a more robust skillset, such as those of a plumber, electrician, carpenter, or handyman.

It is useful to reserve the term "home modifications" to refer to this group of more complex and potentially more expensive projects. Help for special needs homes is available from the local Area Agency on Aging (AAA), the Veterans Administration (VA) and Easter

Seals. Volunteer organizations such as Building Together[12] are also a growing resource.

Home modifications can be reviewed systematically. Because extrinsic risks for falling can be listed by location, it is logical to list the solutions in a similar way. Like hazards, the locations of home modifications for fall risk reduction (sometime referred to as assistive modifications) are be divided into those inside the home and those outside the home (including in the community). Those inside the home can be listed by room. There are user-friendly online sources of information on home modifications, The following list is based largely on the AARP Public Policy Series: *"Aging Friendly" Improvements for Most Every Home Remodeling Project.*[13] It is a list of projects to consider within the context of individual homes and needs.

Home Modifications

THE ENTIRE HOUSE

Raise electrical outlets to 18-24 inches above the floor.

Lower light switches that need to be reached by a wheelchair user.

Change light switches to the rocker/paddle style.

Add motion-sensing automatic light switches as appropriate.

Increase lighting by adding fixtures, but include dimmer switches.

Make doors/doorframes at least 32 inches wide, preferably 36 inches.

Change doorknobs to lever-style hardware.

Install magnetic door stops to hold open doors as needed.

Consider using glowing switch plates and outlet covers that have motion-sensor lights.

STAIRS

Install reliable handrails on both sides of stairwell, anchored into the framing.

Install light switches at the top and bottom of stairwells. (Consider using motion-sensing lights.)

Install electrical outlets at the top and bottom of stairs to permit pathway lighting and to accommodate a possible future stairway chair lift.

Rebuild stairs with stair horizontal depth (tread) of 11 inches (as they are safer than the 10-inch minimum).

Install a chair lift or wheelchair platform lift. These work best with stairs that are 42 inches wide (rather than the standard 36 inches).

Install a ramp for an interior stairway (1-3 steps), or eliminate the stairway by raising the area into which it leads if possible.

BATHROOM

Install grab bars inside and outside the tub or shower, anchored into the framing.

Frame the bathroom with horizontal wood blocking to accommodate installation of grab bars.

Install a pocket door or a barn door, or a hinged door that swings outward at the bathroom entrance, and consider the possibility of using a door handle with no lock.

Create a roll-in shower by rebuilding from scratch or create a zero step-over shower for seated transfer by eliminating the curb. (This requires expert attention to water drainage.)

Install a standard or fold-down bench in the shower area.

Install a sink with wheelchair access, room for legs below with the vanity off to the side.

Install single-lever sink, shower, and bath faucets.

KITCHEN

Counter tops installed at several heights to accommodate both standing and seated use.

Create storage for commonly used list that reduces lifting, reaching, and bending, such as pull-out trays in drawers, and pull-out shelves and baskets in cabinets.

Install automatically closing drawers .

Select and install "age-friendly" appliances such as a stove with front controls, other appliances with well-lighted controls, a refrigerator with side-by-side doors or drawer-style freezer, etc.

Install the dishwasher on an elevated platform to reduce bending and lifting.

Install the microwave at a level that does not demand lifting and stretching (i.e., not above the stove).

Install the sink beside the stove for easy access to put water in a pot or dump hot water out.

Consider a second sink, installed at a lower height with a free area underneath for legs to permit wheelchair or other seated use.

Kitchen sink should have a single-lever faucet .

BEDROOM

Build or rebuild to permit a comfortable first-floor bedroom with access to a bathroom and closet space.

Install low rods and shelves in closets.

Install motion-sensing lights in closets.

Replace bi-fold closet doors with pocket or barn doors to create a wider entrance.

In a build or rebuild situations, locate second-floor closets directly over first-floor closets to facilitate installation of an elevator in the future.

LAUNDRY

Use a motion-sensing light switch because hands are often full.

Select a front-loading washer.

Place shelves and work surfaces at a height that accommodates wheelchair or seated use.

OUTSIDE THE HOME

Ramps can be built in place or premade products can be applied to stairways or elevated thresholds.

Installation of a lifting platform to raise a wheelchair up to a high doorway can be considered.

Building a zero-step entry into the home without a ramp and without permitting water incursion may be possible from a garage.

Assure outside stairs have adequate stair rails — solid, yet small enough to grab, and placed on both sides.

Repair boards in deck areas and consider using non-wood (non-warping) alternatives.

Repair or replace uneven surfaces on walkways, patios, and driveways.

Create shaded areas on outside decks and patios to permit use without overheating during warm weather.

Switch to raised beds in gardening areas.

Home modifications can be expensive. One out of four homes are in need of a substantial assistive modification to prevent falls. According to a survey by the U.S. government in 2008, individuals who need assistive modifications are likely to be older, widowed, non-Hispanic black, on Medicare disability, or are renters.[14] This pattern is unfortunate because home modifications can be expensive.

While grab bars may cost only $150-300, installing a curb-free roll-in shower can be $5000-6000. A full bathroom remodel as much as $9000. Installing multilevel counters in the kitchen is $500-1500, while lowering kitchen cabinets and appliances can be as high as $15,000. A chairlift to the upper story of a home is $3000-4000 and an elevator can be $40,000. The homeowner or landlord is responsible for 80% of these costs and so many projects are left undone — even those of low or moderate cost.[15] Less than 10% of the cost is paid by government programs, even though the government ends up paying billions of dollars each year for fall-related healthcare. This has resulted in the suggestion of paying for reasonably-priced assistive home modifications under Medicare Part D.

What about Medicare for everyone, and for your house? An aspect of the Chronic Care Act passed in the summer of 2018 begins to do just that.

NOTES

[4] *Fall Prevention Research and Practice: A Total Worker Safety Approach to Industrial Health.* 2014 Sep; 52(5): 381–392. doi: 10.2486/indhealth.2014-0110.

[5] Falls Prevention Checklist, Adapted from Temple University's Fall Prevention Project, http://www.networkofcare.org/library/FALLS%20PREVENTION %20CHECKLIS%20Tb.pdf.

[6] Check for Safety: A Home Fall Prevention Checklist, https://www.cdc.gov/ HomeandRecreationalSafety/pubs/English/booklet_Eng_desktop-a.pdf.

[7] Caregiving Checklist: Home Safety, https://assets.aarp.org/external_sites/ caregiving/checklists/checklist_homeSafety.html.

[8] Fall-Proofing Your Home, https://www.nia.nih.gov/health/fall-proofing-your-home.

[9] Mitchell RJ1, Lord SR, Harvey LA, "Associations between obesity and overweight and fall risk, health status and quality of life in older people," Aust N Z J Public Health. 2014 Feb;38(1):13-8. doi: 10.1111/1753-6405.12152.

[10] Home Modification Resource Inventories, http://stopfalls.org/resources/ home-modification-tools-programs-and-funding-landingpage.

[11] Universal Design in Single-Family Housing: A Health Impact Assessment (HIA) in Davidson, NC, https://www.pewtrusts.org/en/~/media/ Assets/2013/11/UniversalDesignandHousinginDavidson,NC.

[12] Building Together, https://rebuildingtogether.org/history.

[13] Aging Friendly' Improvements for Most Every Home Remodeling Project, https://www.aarp.org/livable-communities/housing/info-2016/aging-friendly-renovation-improvements.html)   accessed 8/23/2019.

[14] Home Modifications: Use, Cost, and Interactions with Functioning Among Near-elderly and Older Adults, http://aspe.hhs.gov/daltcp/reports/ 2008/homemod.pdf, accessed 8/23/2019).

[15] Aging in Place Remodeling Costs,(https://www.fixr.com/costs/aging-in-place-remodeling.

CHAPTER 2

INTRINSIC FACTORS

Sometimes I amaze myself at how organized and effective I am, and other times I try to get out of the car with my seatbelt on.

— Anonymous

Falling is not mandatory, but avoiding a fall is not certain in the face of an extrinsic hazard. The outcome at any given moment is a confrontation between the extrinsic hazard and factors intrinsic to the individual. These factors fall into two domains. The first involves the degree of physical skill available to overcome the hazard. This individual intrinsic skill set will be given the name "the functional capacity for not falling."

A strong skill set reduces the risk of falling. Some individuals are burdened by negative aspects of their functional capacity, such as sensory deprivation related to disease or poor vision, and for these people the risk of falling with a given hazard may be amplified. The second domain of intrinsic risk for falling is individual behavior. This can dictate which hazards are confronted. An example of this is insisting upon living alone in an unsafe, although familiar home.

The following discussion of the two domains of intrinsic factors may reference areas of physiology, psychology, and neurological function that will be unfamiliar to many. Certainly, they will be less familiar than the slick floors and loose handrails discussed as extrinsic risk factors in the previous chapter.

The functional capacity for not falling is a skill set that depends upon sensation, power, and attention. These skills, selected through the process of evolution, are then honed through the repetitive trial and error of daily life. Their consolidated effect creates a capacity to not fall. They decline with disuse and with aging. The risk of falling rises as a consequence of this decline in functional capacity. The risk of falling is lessened by improving that functional capacity, or in the case of the elderly, at least slowing the decline.

Behavioral factors can tip the risk of a fall either up or down. Behavior often involves being alert, one of the actual skills at work in the functional capacity for not falling. The behavior of being alert and purposeful raises the functional capacity for not falling. Behaviors such as being inattentive or intoxicated increase the risk of falling. In summary, a fall occurs when this functional capacity for not falling is insufficient to overcome the hazard, when a component of functional capacity amplifies the risk, or when risky behavior raises hazard exposure toward a similar end. Falling due to a hazard is not mandatory, while avoiding a fall is not certain. It all depends on intrinsic factors.

For a neurologist, romance with various obscure complexities of neurophysiology comes easily. How does one organ system coordinate with other organ systems? What is the role of the nervous system? How did it learn to do it? How the brain works and toward what purpose can hold my attention for days. On the other hand, you may be less inclined toward the scientific and hope for some simple recipe — one that is free from opaque terms like "proprioception" and "stochastic resonance," "open-loop feedback," and "neural networks."

Sometimes simple recipes are sufficient, but in this case, not so much. Stay calm. As you enter the tall weeds of neurology in the coming pages, we aspire to clarity for all.

SECTION 1
The Functional Capacity for Not Falling as an Intrinsic Factor

Falling over can be lethal to a tree. While not infused with conscious awareness or fear, a tree expresses a bias for remaining upright. Structural and physiologic features favor success. Oak trees grow with an anchoring mass of roots below ground that are twice the mass of the trunk, branches and leaves above ground. Increasing wind gusts before a hurricane will blow away 30% of the leaves and lush end-branches, thus reducing resistance to the stronger, harsher winds that will follow. Avocado trees simply snap off large brittle branches, while palm trees have the wisdom to bend, offering an indifferent shoulder to the howling wind. Each of these is a tactic that reveals an intrinsic capacity not to fall.

Unlike trees, people stand, strut, prance, and polka. The majority do so without falling even though gravity is unrelenting in its mission to pull us to the ground. The body, composed of a hundred pounds of soft tissue clinging to 206 hinged bones, is a tottering glob perched precariously five to six feet over a ten-toed pedestal. Then it ambles across the room, down the stairs, and out the door. Remarkable.

Successful walking is not due to chance. The patterns of movement to stand and walk without falling flows from a conspiracy of factors — a system. The process is complex and mostly reflexive (pre-conscious). Bones are rigid to bear weight, and hinged or articulated to permit a predictable range of motion. Muscles are aligned to move these bones with precision by contracting and relaxing with calibrated power. In children, the system acquires the skill to walk without falling during routine activities. And over time, the system acquires complex intrinsic capacity for not falling during increasingly complex activities.

Patterns of movement originate from the central nervous system (CNS), the brain, and the spinal cord. Some patterns, like kissing a princess, are conscious, based on intent. Some, like spitting or leaning back from the edge of a cliff, are either intentional or reflexive. Most of the movement that the brain initiates to keep us from falling are pre-conscious reflexive moves that arise from the brain's intrinsic success bias.

The brain initiates an instruction message that is based on intent. It requires prior proprioception, the pre-conscious awareness of posture, and position of the body at the moment the message is initiated. This proprioceptive data is acquired from the sensory system, including data from receptors in joints, and muscles.

In the case of spitting, some of this proprioception comes from the floor of the mouth. These receptors provide data to the brain and the spinal cord, and in a special genius of design, receptors supply data to receptors to make them more or less sensitive. The message is then fine-tuned by the spinal cord, which is armed with its own proprioceptive data. The muscles receive the set of instructions from the CNS and movement occurs.

The system then audits how well the movement achieved the purpose of the message. This is accomplished by monitoring feedback from the sensory nervous system. This instantaneous feedback informs the next instructions from the CNS, and these are therefore increasingly harmonious and effective. Each component of initiating, performing, and then auditing movements is divided into sub-processes.

For example, muscles work as antagonistic pairs across a given joint, with reciprocal contraction and relaxation to produce a finite and predictable response at that joint to a given message. Each component grows more efficient and faster with practice, a process athletes call "motor memory."

An average 10 year-old dreams of being a soccer goalie. She

arrives at practice on day 1, already an accomplished biped. This particular style of gait has served her well for 8 to 9 years. It was acquired over several years with individual effort that built upon CNS pathways learned over thousands of years of trial and error by her species. These lessons are stored in her genes. Her mother is an accomplished biped.

The coach somehow senses that she has a capacity to "grab the ball" and she is told to practice "goalie-awareness" and goalie motor skills and a goalie-feel for the field. Fully attentive to the environment, she hustles to the anticipated site of the next ball grab.

If this is not done well enough, she does skill training for some other position on the team. If, however, she shows promise she trains with drills and games to acquire the reactive "motor memory" that will allow her to be faster and more effective, which will make her a great 10 year-old soccer goalie.

She accumulates balance, power, and purpose to defend the goal against all balls. Every year of practice makes her better and quicker, and she eventually plays for the United States in the Women's World Cup — and wins.

The central nervous system, the sensory nervous system, and the muscles together learn to create effective countermeasures to the pull of gravity. They function as a single coordinated high-speed entity — a system. Each part is intricate. The overall system is complex.

In order to efficiently discuss how any system works, how it fails, and what to do about that failure, that system must be given a name. In a sport called "Not Falling," the name of that system will be "The Functional Capacity for Not Falling." Balance, power, and purpose will be the pillars upon which it rests.

A name "Not Falling System" seems absurd on the surface. The mandatory consumption of food is not called "The Not Starvation System." It is called eating. The capacity to speak without spitting is not called "The No Spittle System." We are not sure what to call it.

But falling is a more intense and moment-to-moment risk than starvation or drooling. It uniformly demands a system that robustly functions within milliseconds in order to be successful, as in the 10 year-old soccer star. A discussion designed to reduce falls in the elderly is well-served by giving this functional capacity this oppositional name, and understanding its elements.

The Pillars of the Functional Capacity for Not Falling

The set of sensory, motor and cognitive skills that form the basis for the functional capacity for not falling is supported on three pillars. The first is *balance*. The second pillar is *power*. The third is *purpose*.

Balance, power, and purpose are each an inherited set of skills. Each is nourished by training and diminished by neglect. Each is a functional capacity made up of an underlying set of skills.

Balance is made up of vestibular (middle ear) skill , visual skills, and a sensory skill called "proprioception." Power is the consequence of skillful muscle contraction under the complex control of the spinal cord, brainstem, and brain. Purpose sets the goal and is sub-served by the cognitive skills sets of attention, intention, and attitude.

The first pillar, balance, is often viewed as predominantly a vestibular skill set. In reality, the key essential building block of balance rests elsewhere. Balance can only be understood by exploring proprioception. This is the sense of the position of the body with reference to the world around it, as well as the sense of the position of one part of the body with reference to another part.

It is sometimes called the "sixth sense." It not only perceives the position of the body in space but also senses how that position is changing. Proprioception registers and processes the position and movement of joints, muscles, and skin. It also audits the relative position of objects and self in visual space by processing data registered by the eye. Additionally, proprioception processes position change as identified by kinetic displacements of the head as recognized by the vestibular apparatus of the middle ear.

This becomes a river of proprioceptive data, much of which escapes conscious recognition. Subconscious processing of this data in the brain and in the spinal cord centers triggers responses in other body systems, such as muscles. These responses are themselves fine-tuned when this unending stream of proprioception transmits new updated positional data.

For example, when proprioception perceives that the left foot has slipped rapidly forward on the wet floor, weight is urgently shifted to the right foot and the body remains upright. Then the weight is shifted back to both feet. Proprioception informs a rapid guided application of power to successfully achieve its purpose: balance.

The middle ear does its job with fluid filled channels which mirror the position of the head relative to the pull of gravity. It transforms kinetic mechanical data into electrical impulses in a process referred to as "transduction." These impulses are continuously transmitted to central processing centers in the brainstem (the lower portion of the brain) which decipher the data and are thereby informed about a change of position.

With regard to the eye, the retina "sees" objects and creates electrical impulses imprinted with the changing spatial relationships between these objects. These impulses constantly arrive at central processing centers in the brain and brainstem, adding to proprioception.

Probably the most robust source of proprioception are "mechanoreceptors." The role of mechanoreceptors in fall risk reduction is rich in opportunity for innovative thinking. Most people have never heard of them.

Mechanoreceptors are microscopic clusters of cells within skin, muscles, and joints. They have been named in a chaotic fashion. In the skin, position-sensing receptors sensitive to stretch or pressure are named according to their speed and sensitivity (slow adapting versus rapid adapting).

They send tactile information which is informative about position change to the brain, brainstem, and spinal cord. Specialized clusters of cells within the muscle tissue are called "muscle spindles." They generate electrical signals in response to being stretched or shortened.

"Golgi Tendon Apparatus" (GTA) is the name given to a similar structure within tendons which function in much the same way. They both send data-rich electrical impulses to the brain, the brainstem, and the spinal cord. Informative signals from muscle spindles and GTA are then distributed to many areas including those in muscles that pull in the opposite direction.

One brilliant aspect of evolution, touched upon earlier, is that muscle spindles and GTA send messages to themselves. This causes an adjustment to their sensitivity, permitting their data to be reliable through a very broad range of stretching or shortening. This is, in some ways, similar to the dilation or constriction of the pupil to preserve the sensitivity of the retina over a broad range of lighting.

In addition to skin and muscle mechanoreceptors, there are receptors in joints and in the ligaments surrounding joints. These are called "free nerve endings," "Rufini endings," and "Pacini corpuscles." These register tissue deformation and joint angular displacement creating a sensory skill called "kinesthesia." This data is distributed broadly in a fashion similar to muscle spindles and GTA.

Maintaining or changing body position involves lots of skin, muscle, tendon, and joint receptors. The subsequent proprioceptive "river of data" is a rich source of information. It monitors small and large changes in position with both sensitivity and specificity. It is a system of data acquisition and internal feedback that exceeds the complexity of many other central nervous system functions.

The river of proprioceptive data flows slowly in a newborn. It picks up speed through infancy and childhood as new pathways come into use through a maturation process of "myelination," — the laying down of an insulating goop that makes neurological pathways carry data faster. New sources of information are then trained by tasks that are repeated. Then, with repetition and trial and error, proprioception gains the capacity to briskly answer the questions: where is the body, where is it going and at what rate?

When proprioception falters due to illness or aging, these questions are answered less well and the functional capacity for not falling declines. The hopeful note is that even in disease or late in life, proprioception can respond to training. That is why mechanoreceptors and proprioception provide an opportunity for innovative thinking. And, now you have heard them.

The second pillar, power, is the component of the functional capacity for not falling that allows an active physical response to a circumstance once that circumstance has been identified by proprioception. Power permits the body to achieve a purpose. This power can be static or dynamic. Static power retains a posture in a static environment. Dynamic power retains posture in a changing environment, or attains a new intended posture.

Power may be sufficient or insufficient for any of these tasks. It is generated by muscles acting on skeletal structures. As with the aspects of balance, muscular power is an inherited functional capacity. It is nourished by training (exercise) and diminished by neglect. The loss of muscular power among aging individuals is highly variable but common. A loss due to aging or disease can improve with exercise or worsen further with neglect.

Power is not uniform. Individuals do not inherit the same potential and do not train it to the same degree. Muscle tissue is composed of fibers of several different biochemical types. "Slow twitch" type 1 fibers are best suited for protracted effort, and "fast twitch" type 2 fibers for sudden effort.

The relative number of each fiber type varies between people. Athletes who successfully run sprints often have paradoxically large and well defined upper body musculature. It is not just because they lift weights. They were born with, or they have nurtured, a predominance of fast twitch fibers. This fiber type favors fast running for short distances, and this fiber type tends to hypertrophy quite nicely with use.

Fast twitch fibers are used by a person who is about to fall, perceives this impending fall subconsciously by proprioception, and then initiates a fast and effective corrective power response. It has been noted under the microscope that the number of type 2 fast twitch fibers decline with age. However, appropriate exercises can significantly slow this process,

Purpose is the third pillar of the functional capacity for not falling. Much of purpose has to do with the conscious and pre-conscious ingrained nature of the human brain. It is imbued by evolution and experience with a success bias. Not falling is success.

Success is increased by have not falling as a goal and attention to risk as a strategy. "Be careful to not fall." Sage advice. A simple reminder to anyone, including older adults.

The specifics of what to do in order to "be careful" are undefined. It is reminiscent of Smokey Bear who famously said, "Only you can prevent forest fires." The message is enhanced by the attention grabbing presence of a carnivore in a hat, but it is the suggestion of individual responsibility that really carries the message.

Perhaps signs with a new messenger, "Schmegegy the Goose" (an herbivore in a kilt), should be posted throughout the community saying: "Only You Can Be Careful Not to Fall."

Despite some obvious virtues, this tactic probably tumbles headlong into the simplicity trap. H.L. Mencken reminded us, "For every complex problem there is a simple solution which is probably incorrect." After all, kids continue to speak with food in their mouth, residents litter under penalty of law, and not everyone elects to just say no. Purpose is not a slogan on a poster. It is a mind-set with separate skill components that can be individually addressed.

In early years, a child at play will often fall and scrape something. Knees get cut repeatedly, but most kids will only cut their chin once. The chin event provokes a conscious purpose and a pre-conscious preference not to do it again. The purpose and preference is accomplished by the application of skills identified as "attention, intention, and attitude."

On each play day, proprioception and power are trained by pre-conscious purpose. This continues for many years. Proprioception and power are permissive and supportive, but it is purpose that milks the cow or climbs the ladder. The capacity to pursue these things without falling results from the honed skills for attention, intention, and attitude. Much like the functional capacity for running with speed and endurance, these are skills that become better through training. And they get worse through neglect — and aging.

Attitude, a component of purpose, is a determinant of fall risk. Attitude is a settled way of thinking that is reflected in behavior. It can arise from personal experience or witnessing the experiences of others, or it may emerge full-cloth from one's personality. Attitudes are nouns like nihilism, stubbornness, vanity, negativism, and indifference, just to name a few.

But each gains additional meaning as an adjective. For example, he is stubborn. They appear to be indifferent. Sometimes a choice is "just because," — an impulsive choice. More commonly it is the predictable and repeated expression of an attitude. If such a choice leads to poor exercise, bad nutrition, reduced social interaction or even dangerous behaviors, then the risk of falls increases. Attitude cannot be neglected as a risk for falling. An attitude that embraces daily exercise can have quite the opposite effect.

Fear is an example of an attitude that can have a significant impact on the risk of falling. Some fears result from realistic anxiety in anticipation of an adverse event. Fear behaviors, such as caution in the face of a hazard, can be a positive strategy.

Conversely, other fear motivated behaviors can be harmful. Fear of falling can cause muscles to tighten at the first sign of a fall, increasing the overall likelihood of falling as well as the severity of related injuries. Fear of being identified as a person who falls is an intrinsic risk factor that cuts across many other areas of concern. Fear of falling and fear of being identified as someone who falls reduces physical activity. Proprioception, power, and purpose are all adversely affected by fear because each is diminished with inactivity.

Furthermore, reduced physical activity leads to reduced social activity. Then, in turn, this breeds poor self-esteem, isolation, depression, and loneliness (also attitudes), which are independently associated with increased risk for fall-related injury. Fear and depression lead to a counter-productive excessive focus on the area of deficiency, such as weak muscles rather than on the constructive focus to compensate with more exercise.

Society sends negative signals about a person who falls. They should not be left alone, live alone, or even think independently. These societal attitudes are meant to engender safety, but often become part of the problem.

Anyone can step on a child's toy and if balance and attention are good it is an unremarkable event. It can be a painful and disruptive fall if balance or attention are insufficient. In a society inclined to shame them, older-age adults with reduced intrinsic capacity might fall and then shift the blame for the fall, insisting and believing that the toy was the sole culprit. The true situation is denied.

Anticipated loss of self-esteem becomes more compelling than the alternate, more reasonable fear, that unnecessary falls will follow — again, if the true situation is denied. Denial can even lead to a defensive claim that "it never happened."

Failure to report falls may also be an aspect of fear or other attitude, such as anger, frustration, or stubbornness. It is both intuitive and analytically correct to conclude that reducing environmental hazards is an appropriate strategy to reduce falls. It is all the more necessary to do so in the face of reduced intrinsic capacity, especially when there is fear and denial.

Attention and intention, two requisite components of purpose, are related determinants of fall risk. Adequate attention to an extrinsic hazard permits an effective volitional application of power, or it triggers appropriate reflexive acts, and the intentional act meets with success. Insufficient attention is a generalized behavior that is an impediment to the functional capacity for not falling. The lack of willful intent to avoid risk under a circumstance of increased risk is another aspect of purpose, and as such, an area of intrinsic risk for falling.

It is conventional wisdom that people will make a robust effort to avoid falling. This is incorrect (as conventional wisdom is often incorrect). Inadequate conscious intent to avoid falling is common. This can be due to distraction from a single "sparkly" event across the room or perhaps when a person attends to three events in an environment where four events are happening concurrently.

She may not be able to sustain an intention to avoid risk if she walks and carries a package and hears a siren and steps off a curb all at the same time. Intoxication can bring poor balance and disrupts attention. A drunk intent on hiking to Bavaria will probably be inattentive to the fall risk posed by the doorsill of the pub.

Dementing illness is similar. A person with dementia who fails to acknowledge weakness, neglects a visual impairment, or wanders inattentively, will fall. Reduction in cognitive capacity and inattention can also occur due to sleep deprivation, depression, recreational drugs, and combinations of various pharmaceutical agents.

A cumulative decline in functional capacity will reflect any net decline among the three pillars. Each of the components (balance, power, purpose) may vary independent of the other.

The relationship between a decline and the risk for falling is non-linear. That is, the functional capacity for not falling does not decline, or improve, by finite increments. What we see is the proverbial scenario of "the straw that broke the camel's back." A person might do well-enough despite a partial decline in functional capacity. Falls are thus avoided. Then the decline reaches a point of "sufficient insufficiency," the tipping point, after which falls occur — and recur.

SECTION 2
Behavior as in Intrinsic Factor

Some behaviors flow from natural patterns of life and introduce predictable patterns of risk. For example, people with good balance sometimes fall. It tends to occur in a community setting, at places where circumstances are variable and demanding, such as stepping off the escalator at a busy mall.

People with less balance or moderately reduced "Functional Capacity" fall most often in and about the home. Even though the hazards in the home are more predictable and uniform than those encountered in the community, these mildly compromised individuals spend more time inside the home than out and about. Home is where they are most likely to attempt independent behaviors, such as stepping out of the shower. Falls in the yard and garage are far more common in men than in women due to gender-based differences in behaviors. People with poor balance and poor functional capacity sometimes actually fall less than their contemporaries because they attempt fewer independent activities than their less-severely afflicted counterparts.

Many behavioral patterns arise as part of the warp and woof of personality. A "couch potato" is a good person who prefers to avoid exercise, and by this behavior reduces their functional capacity for not falling. People often fail to exercise out of benign intent, such as perceived physical restraints, time limitations, or social and cultural barriers.

"Exercise well, balance well" can get lost in the shuffle. A person might fail to accept the virtues of exercise or reducing environmental hazards if they are indifferent by nature, or if they have been rendered so by an attitude of denial.

Some behaviors reveal a covert form of denial — the failure to be sufficiently "risk adverse." If an 80-year-old continues to climb a ladder, the best solution is to hide the ladder.

Falling with the intention of doing so does occur in persons with dependency needs in search of help. Hopefully, these falls cause only minimal bodily harm and allow the identification of people with unmet needs to be recognized and responded to thoughtfully.

Some behavioral patterns are more sinister. Alcoholism is a

behavioral pattern common to millions of Americans. Among the many aspects of alcoholism is the tendency to increase risky behaviors and to fall more. Specific alcohol-induced health issues can involve the pillars of the functional capacity for not falling. Proprioception declines during intoxication and after years of alcohol's toxic effect on nerves and reflexes. Power is reduced as muscles atrophy in the face of reduced exercise, poor nutrition, and systemic decline. Attention, intention, and attitude are eroded. Risky behaviors confront environmental hazards with blunted capacity and covert denial.

Medications can also increase falling. The pattern of alcoholism is replicated in those who abuse sedatives or narcotic medications. But, some sensitive individuals can have an increased fall risk after even a single dose of a medication to which they have a unique sensitivity. Some drugs that are well-tolerated in most people might cause recurrent falls in an individual with low blood pressure. Medications that are benign may become intolerable when taken in combination with other medications or conspire with alcohol. These effects can be sneaky.

Behaviors that lead to falls should be modified to reduce the risk. This can be as simple as just doing it and as difficult as one could possibly imagine. Giving up smoking is an example of this, and there is robust literature about AIDS prevention, alcohol abstinence and workplace safety that testify to how difficult behavioral change for risk reduction can be.

According to Plato, human behavior flows from three main sources: desire, emotion, and knowledge. Behavior in aging may be an exception. With aging comes limitations and with limitations comes loss of self-esteem and the indignities of the loss of autonomy. These then dictate attitude and intent. The category of behavior that occurs when beach flip-flops trigger a fall in an 85 year-old is not easily assigned to issues of knowledge, desire, or emotion. With all due respect to Plato, the choice of these ill-fitting shoes flows from mindless habit.

The checklist for intrinsic factors is shorter than the one for the extrinsic factors. Regrettably, the identified responses are often less easily achieved. The following checklist is not so much an activity as it is a thought exercise.

Checklist For Intrinsic Factors For Fall Risk Reduction

☐ Medical conditions present or uncertain?

☐ Make an appointment with your physician to assure that conditions that might lead to falling are fully diagnosed and properly managed. This may include, but not be limited to neurological, cardiac, orthopedic, arthritic, or middle ear disorders. **Report actual falls or fall concerns.**

☐ Muscle weakness disorders from inactivity, chronic disease, medications, primary disorders of muscles, low thyroid.

- ☐ Loss of sensation from alcoholism, diabetes, or neuropathy.

- ☐ Low blood pressure from medications, dehydration, neuropathy or cardiac disorders. Low blood pressure on standing for no clear reason (Primary Autonomic Failure — PAF).

- ☐ Disordered walking from stroke, Parkinson's disease, orthopedic or arthritic conditions.

- ☐ Poor vision (see below).

- ☐ Balance disorder from Middle Ear, low blood pressure, loss of sensation, disordered vision, medication adverse effects

- ☐ Disorder of alertness and attention related to medications, alcoholism, liver, renal, or endocrine gland disorders, memory disorders.

☐ Current medications have the lowest risk of falls?

- ☐ Ask your physician to confirm that you are taking the best medications for your condition in the context of fall risk reduction.

- ☐ Confirm that you are taking all medications as instructed and if not, be sure to do so.

- ☐ If you have more than one physician, confirm that all pertinent information is shared and that each one is aware of your full medication list.

- ☐ Ask your physician to review potential interactions if you are on two or more medications.

☐ Ask your physician to review any dizziness or light-headed sensations in the specific context of a possible medication-adverse event to which an elderly patient might be more sensitive than a younger one.

☐ Your pharmacist is a reliable source of advice regarding medication side effects and interactions.

☐ Eye conditions that could cause a fall fully managed?

☐ Ask your eye doctor to confirm proper prescription for glasses.

☐ Ask your eye doctor to diagnose and treat cataracts or glaucoma if necessary.

☐ Intrinsic capacity for not falling suspected of being insufficient or in decline?

☐ Improve balance, power, and purpose by working with a physical therapist, occupational therapist, or physical trainer. This may require a physician referral.

☐ Improve balance, power, and purpose by working on your own. Guidance is available online, via YouTube, through subscription services, and in printed programs from both private and public agencies.

☐ Improve balance, power, and purpose by participating in a community-based exercise program that has evidence-based success in falls prevention.

☐ Have you fallen doing something stupid or unnecessary?

☐ Seek help with your behavior from a psychologist or a trusted friend, clergy, or community agency if it involves drug and alcohol use.

☐ Pay attention to the potential negative consequences of risky activities at home or in the yard, and let that guide you on a less painful path.

☐ Consider changing a "societal behavior" such as moving to an assisted-living facility or into the residence of a family member for health or safety reasons.

☐ Give your ladder to a youthful neighbor.

SECTION 3
Societal Behavior Modification: Leaving Home

Much of what is known about extrinsic risks in the environment has been accumulated rather than scientifically discovered. The tactics used have been observation and intuition. Critical analysis has often been limited to a "necessary afterthought." This tactic proves useful in the creation of a checklist of extrinsic factors for falling.

However, these tactics have not always served us so well. An important failure of intuition occurred when we were confronted with what to do with advanced-age adults who had declined beyond their capacity to remain home alone, and we decided to put them in nursing homes.

Over the last 80 years, American culture has reversed an earlier trend to care for aged relatives at home. Multi-generational households have become scarce. In addition, birth control in the modern era has widened the age gap between elderly parents and their children. The female reproductive interval, which used to end at menopause (45-55 years of age), now effectively ends by age 40.

Prior to 1940, a 70-year-old partially disabled adult was likely to have an 18-year-old child still at home. Now that same impaired 70-year-old has a youngest child who is 30 years old, with two kids and a home of her own. Intuition said that in this setting, in the face of a decline in functional capacity, the best alternative to staying in the "risky home" was to move a vulnerable person into a safe facility with nurses and nurse's aides — a nursing home. Sensible? Not so much as it seemed at first.

All too often, the loss of a beloved home produced depression and reduced self-esteem. The loss of autonomy bred hopelessness. The loss of familiar surroundings fostered poor cognition. The removal from the society of neighbors and the familiarity of community leads to isolation. All of these lead to inactivity, and a resultant worsening in all categories. The unfortunate history of nursing home placement is that many of the vulnerabilities went unchecked. Poor nutrition continued, falls recurred. Memory declined. Frailty worsened. While the family accrued a small gain in comfort and hope, the elderly client is the one who paid a high price.

The sciences of architecture and social engineering have created the more modern-era assisted-living facility (ALF). Compared to a limited function nursing home, the ALF environment is better designed to preserve the dignity of its residents. This has had a downstream consequence of preserving the functional capacity for not falling in some facilities.

There are many variations in the size and structure of an ALF. A larger facility allows a resident to enter the system at a level that meets their need. "Independent living," by example, might be an apartment with housekeeping and meals provided. The general environment could include an array of art and history classes, group fitness programs, game rooms, and organized day trips — all designed to increase socialization, foster wellness, improve balance, support self-esteem, and in the process, these can help reduce falling.

Such facilities often offer basic healthcare. Smaller group homes are less likely to offer as many activities, but they can offer more personal interaction. As functional capacity declines over the course of several years, a resident in an ALF might change to an assisted-living apartment, or move to a new ALF with assisted-living capacity.

An assisted-living apartment generally offers many of the same features as in independent-living facilities, but will characteristically also supply assistance which includes daily hygiene, and a nurse to administer daily meds. Many larger facilities have skilled nursing or rehab units, or memory disorder units for those who, temporarily or persistently, are no longer suited for assisted living.

There are many iterations of the concept, and they are evolving.

The ALF concept is a clear improvement over the "warehousing" feel of nursing homes of previous decades. An ALF works to reduce the social and emotional hardship of leaving home, and this is associated with fewer falls. The average cost of an ALF is $48,000 per year.[16]

SECTION 4
Societal Behavior Modification: Staying Home

Between 50 and 80% (references vary) of late-age adults volunteer that they would prefer to stay in their own home forever. Some agree to leave only under coercion. I know of two who left only after the house burned down. Behavior modification is not necessary to get them to stay, but is necessary in order to get them to do so safely. Social scientists, along with home modification architects and local policy makers, have been working for years on an alternative lifestyle called "Aging in Place."[17, 18] The goal is to permit advanced-age adults to remain in their home by creating the necessary support networks.

A proper Aging in Place program can be associated with fewer falls, lower healthcare costs, and better health than if these same individuals had stayed in their home without proper modifications, or had had moved into a nursing home. Statistics suggest it is better than an ALF, and over several years it is measurably less expensive. And with fewer falls, costs drop significantly for Medicare,

Medicaid, and community agencies.[19]

Fall rates relate to behaviors. Socialization, regular exercise, proper healthcare and eye care, good nutrition, and wearing proper foot gear all reduce the risk for falling. Consuming alcohol or climbing on a chair to reach a high shelf all increase the risk of falling. Behavioral adjustment requires the elderly adult to "buys in" and participate.

Not falling is clearly better than falling, but not everyone is paying attention. Participation is enhanced when it is viewed as the best way for someone to stay in their own home. That's part of the secret sauce — the chance to do whatever they prefer to do. Also, many will participate in changing their behaviors because they view aging in place as cost-effective, even though this can be hard to prove. Aging in place needs this attitude of participation, but a successful program requires attention to two areas of concern.

First, the process incurs expense. The built environment must be modified to meet the needs of the elderly by performing a checklist audit of the home in order to reduce hazards and by applying the lessons of Universal Design. Correction of hazards can sometimes be expensive. Significant home modifications can cost thousands of dollars. Costs are relative and must be viewed in the context of alternative costs.

Falls hurt and can produce fear and depression, and sometimes result in significant direct healthcare costs. Fall-related disability will increase the cost of home health aides or even lead to need to move out of the home to an (expensive) ALF or skilled-nursing facility. Many of the direct and secondary costs of falls are born by Medicare, Medicaid, or other public and private programs. Advisory panels are considering the wisdom of funding home modifications that prevent falls through these health-related agencies.[20]

Second, a healthcare and exercise support network is necessary. If it does not exist, it must be created. Communities must provide safe streets to ensure "walkability." Advocates for the aged need to support an environment that enables life-long exercise, sustained social interactions, counseling, and medical support. Community-sponsored group exercise programs that are evidence-based (proven to reduce falls by a scientific randomized controlled study) can be initiated with the assistance of local healthcare organizations and the Area Agency on Aging. These might include Tai Chi, A Matter of Balance, CAPABLE, Healthy Steps for Older Adults, or multifaceted programs like Stepping On. The National Council on Aging (NCOA) is a robust resource for these.[21]

A social support network is also necessary and must be created if it does not exist. Retirement communities have found favor among many aging baby boomers. They come for the golf course and the pool, and for the opportunity to give up lawn maintenance. And they make this move hoping to find their forever home where they can age in place These communities often have the corporate wisdom to include programs for social networking, exercise groups, access to healthcare and shopping, assisted transportation, and the incorporation of Universal Design. Unfortunately, the majority of these communities are beyond the financial means of many Americans.

There are retirement communities that simply develop without specific planning. Many elderly adults still live in the multifamily dwellings that they first occupied when raising their families. Forty years ago there were children. Now the children are grown and gone and the elderly parents have stayed on. The multifamily dwelling has become a "Naturally Occurring Retirement Community" (NORC).[22] This is a form of aging in place.

Hazard modification is critically important as these are often old buildings. Home modifications are no less needed in this group than in a single family house in an upscale suburb, but cost barriers can be daunting. On a positive note, with many people living in one area, healthcare, social, and transportation needs may more easily be met by community-based programs.

There are creative strategies to avoid moving from a conventional home into an institution-like ALF. The simplest form involves neighbors sharing tasks. A young neighbor takes care of shopping for food and checking in on an elderly man next door, who in turn provides after-school supervision for the younger neighbor's kids.

In a more complex relationship, 10-20 elderly households may join, with the help of a community-based social services agency, to function as a village in order to assist each other. Some places have constructed such "senior villages," and there are "village-to-village networks" to help do it right.[23] A "Co-housing Project" is an organized relationship of elderly individuals living in private homes with a common house that includes a kitchen for preparing communal meals, social areas, and also extra housing for guests and caregivers.[24]

The behavioral modification of staying at home has gained the attention of local policy makers. Zoning, planning, and transportation decisions are increasingly designed to insure safe neighborhoods that have "walkability," and to support the creation of satisfactory low-cost areas with access to transportation and shopping so that the elderly can age in place.

NOTES

[16] How Much does Assisted Living Cost, https://www.whereyoulive matters.org/how-much-does-assisted-living-cost/accessed 8/24/2019.

[17] Sarinnapha Vasunilashorn,1 Bernard A. Steinman, Phoebe S. Liebig, and Jon Pynoos, "Aging in Place: Evolution of a Research Topic Whose Time Has Come," *Journal of Aging Research*, Volume 2012, Article ID 120952, 6 pages.

[18] Aging in Place: Growing Older at Home, https://www.nia.nih.gov/health/aging-place-growing-older-home.

[19] Older Adult Falls - Costly But Not Inevitable, https://www.healthaffairs.org/do/10.1377/hblog20180402.25780/full/.

[20] Overcoming Obstacles To Policies For Preventing Falls By The Elderly: FINALREPORT, https://www.hud.gov/sites/documents/OVERCOMINGOBSTACLESFALLS.PDF.

[21] Exercise Programs that Promote Senior Fitness, https://www.ncoa.org/center-for-healthy-aging/basics-of-evidence-based-programs/physical-activity-programs-for-older-adults/.

[22] Bedney, B. J., Goldberg, R. B., & Josephson, K. (2010). "Aging in place in naturally occurring retirement communities: Transforming aging through supportive service programs," *Journal of Housing for the Elderly*, 24(3–4), 304–321.

[23] Village to Village Network: What is a Village, https://www.vtvnetwork.org/.

[24] Creating Neighborhood One Community at a Time, https://www.cohousing.org.

CHAPTER 3
THINGS THAT GO BUMP IN THE FUTURE

"Speculation is never a waste of time. It clears away the deadwood in the thickets of deduction."

— Elizabeth Peters, He Shall Thunder in the Sky

Observation, intuition and scientific analysis are tools that form the tactical basis for understanding fall prevention. They give perspective to the past, inform the present, and indicate pathways for the future. Speculation is a tool. It embodies more than guesswork or conjecture. It contains a notion of genius based on the sense that "the past is prologue to the future," a prelude that gestures to where substantial gains will lie. It is this prospect of substantial gains that animates meaningful speculation.

SECTION 1
Proprioception in Physical Therapy

Patients of all types receive physical therapy (PT). When the patient has an illness or an injury that includes a physical impairment that is expected to get better with time, PT is offered to shorten the time and maximize the recovery. If an individual is expected to remain the same, PT is designed to maximize safety and independence for the activities of daily living. The elderly are often viewed as afflicted — as having a condition that is anticipated to invariably worsen. Their PT is often offered to minimize harm and delay the inevitable. When this tyranny of low expectations is applied to PT in the elderly, it may result in a woeful underestimation of what is possible. With more attention to the role of proprioception, PT for fall prevention in the elderly can be more robust, and may "maximize recovery."

Conventional therapy for fall prevention is generally directed at static balance, flexibility, and agility. PT includes muscle strengthening, stretching, aerobic exercises, and health education. Usual activities involve marching in place, knee lifts, heel digs, shoulder rolls, knee bends, and stretching of the major muscle groups.

Exercises are gradually increased in difficulty over time on an individual basis. However, an enlightened extension of PT with a proprioceptive perspective will focus on static balance with squats or one leg standing. Exercises for dynamic balance will include jogging back and forth on a short course, sideways walking, forward walking in a zigzag line, and backward walking. There might be transitions between postures while performing functional everyday movements, not unlike Tai Chi. Understanding why these work for the elderly will lead to better therapies in the future.

Proprioceptive signals from mechanoreceptors weaken with age.

Transduction from muscle spindles become less intense with weakness and atrophy of the muscle tissue. Mechanoreceptor age-related disease is not yet described but almost certainly happens. Signal weakness is worsened by diseases of peripheral nerves that must carry the signal from the receptors to the brain and spinal cord centers. The effect of these weakened signals is further blunted by slowed processing at these centers. The resulting postural reflexes are ineffective. Spatial and temporal defects then open the door to falls. The obvious treatment for this is to increase the sensitivity of the mechanoreceptors, reverse the dysfunction of peripheral nerves, reverse the blunted response in central processing centers, and reduce the defects in postural reflexes — or some combination of all these things.

With regard to increasing the signal from mechanoreceptors, muscle spindles are a major contributor to the proprioceptive data stream. Their sensitivity is being set and reset on a regular basis during muscle activity throughout life. This modulation is under the control of what are called "alpha neurons."

These have nerve fibers that travel from the spinal cord to the spindles. These alpha neurons are active when there is physical activity on a regular basis and are less easily activated during intervals of prolonged inactivity. This is the result of a specific differential gene expression in the spinal cord centers. Prolonged inactivity dictates reduced alpha neuron activity, which leads to reduced sensitivity of the muscle spindle, which leads to weakened proprioceptive signals, and thus falls. The reversal of this process occurs with a return to physical activity. The theory, supported by research, is that exercise causes an alternate gene to be expressed[25] which leads to increased alpha neuron activity. Stronger proprioceptive signal from the muscle spindle follows, as does fewer falls.

With regard to reversing the weakness of peripheral nerves, this is possible but not probable. It is generally limited to a few clinical circumstances such as a B12 or thiamine deficiency (which can be measured with simple blood tests). Reduced alcohol consumption and management of metabolic conditions, helped by exercise, can keep dysfunction from worsening. The participation of an internal medicine physician might help prevent falls by rescuing peripheral nerve function.

With regard to speeding the function of aging spinal cord centers, these centers function under the direction of genetic foci within their DNA. Some slowing of function that occurs in aging is cellular and may be unavoidable. Some slowing is the expression of a different gene site than that which was expressed in earlier more active years. This genetic expression of a "younger" gene can be induced by exercises, especially exercises that are varied and multiplanar.[25] Proprioceptive data processing is viewed as trainable by specific proprioceptive exercise that bombard the centers with proprioceptive data that demands processing. This can reduce falls.

With regard to reducing the defects in postural reflexes, these reflexes provoke rapid forceful muscle contraction. A mechanoreceptor called the "Golgi tendon apparatus" (GTA) blocks signals that trigger forceful muscle contraction when the GTA senses that the tendon is not ready-and-able to handle the forceful event. Regular physical activity, including stretching, can cause the GTI to be more permissive. Postural reflexes then become more effective with fewer falls. Physical activity that includes proper stretching reduces falls

New things are being added. Exercises initially done on one foot while holding the back of a chair can now advance to unsteady surfaces like a balance board, or the Bosu Ball.[26] These can then give way to a variably unsteady treatment platform, like the Pedalo Stabilizer, which permits multi-sensory training.[27]

For those who "....have fallen and can't get up," buttons on a pendant can give way to wearable accelerometers and video surveillance systems that identify a fall even without an active report by the person who has fallen. The prediction of fall risk has depended on clinical evaluation, but new wearable devices, video capture systems, force plate platforms, and sensors implanted in walkways can quantify postural reflexes producing a targeted balance assessment.[28]

Therapists can test vision and middle ear function and other proprioceptive components independently. They can measure the response to perturbations (rapid unanticipated displacements) of the base and this then segregates deficits, such as delayed compensation versus over-compensation, into treatment categories. Virtual reality (VR) systems can now create a stress environment during any training situation.

This systematic attention to proprioception will grow as we become more familiar with evolving research. Robust diagnostic and therapeutic opportunities may arise when the primary disorders of mechanoreceptor are better understood. Until that happens, the incremental application of newer technology is welcome.

SECTION 2
The Benefit Of Segmentation

Entities must not be multiplied beyond necessity.

— William of Occam

"When you hear hoof beats behind you, expect to see a horse and not a zebra."

"Rob the bank because that is where the money is."

"If it ain't broke don't fix it."

These pithy aphorisms embody guidance first offered by a Franciscan friar, William of Occam, in the 13th century. The following aphorism is referred to as "Occam's Razor:" "When facing a choice between several causes, select the cause that has the fewest variables."

It is not a rule. It is a heuristic, a "rule of thumb," a way of thinking. When this method of thinking is applied to medicine it can be very helpful.

A man with both a swollen calf and shortness of breath may have a dangerous condition. He should be evaluated for a possible blood clot to his lung (pulmonary embolism) from a leg vein condition (thrombophlebitis), even though, his leg and his lung may be two unrelated conditions. We can add to the dilemma of solving problems well the wisdom of H.L. Mencken, who said, "For every complex problem there is a solution that is clear, simple, and wrong."

Occam's Razor can lead to errors when applied to something complicated, like healthcare. An alternate heuristic was offered in the 20th century by Dr John Hickum. Referred to as "Hickum's Dictum," it states, "A man can have as many diseases as he damn well pleases." For example, the man with the swollen leg may have been kicked by a horse and his shortness of breath may be an allergic reaction to horse manure.

How does all of this relate to fall prevention? The preceding chapters have outlined categories of risks for falling, categories from which to select the villainous cause. How we think is important in this selection process.

It is 7:00 A.M., 14 hours since Dr. Jones first parked her 10-year-old Corvette behind the outpatient clinic and walked to the emergency room to begin her shift. She can hear the familiar fatigue in her voice. Her empathy remains intact. It has been 44 patients and 44 charts and two deaths. It has been people with an honest urgent need, and a few people without an urgent need — but with an evident preference for the place. And there were five falls. Each fall came to the ER out of concern: "Do I have a serious injury? Why did it happen? Will I fall again?"

"Concern" is the preferred word of a tired doctor. For the layperson, the word is "fear." Fear and uncertainty is far more intense than concern — and fear may have actually been the "cause with the fewest variables" in some of the patients.

She asked each of them why they fell and reviewed the circumstance to find a most likely single cause. She knew that identifying the proximate cause offered the best opportunity to avoid a recurrence. Asking how it happened was mandatory.

Sometimes a finite cause was identified, but often the answers were uninformative. "I slipped. I tripped. I don't know. I felt it coming. I never felt it coming. I found myself on the floor."

The cause recorded by her in the chart? "Multi-factorial." Data without information made each case seem uniquely complex — too complex to resolve in an ER visit. Dr Jones asked the question and tried to listen to the answer, and then, when possible, she sent them home with a falls prevention pamphlet that included 12 recommendations on how to avoid the next visit to the ER.

Regrettably, fear is not an emotion that is easily subdued, even by the assurances of a qualified physician and an informative pamphlet.

Complex circumstances are clarified by information. The complexity of causes for an acute fall can be addressed the same way as the complexity of organizing and navigating a grocery store: by creating categories with segmentation that send a person down the right aisle. It is this strategy of segmentation which allows us to successfully feed, clothe, and shelter ourselves in a world of mind-boggling alternatives and shifting barriers to progress.

Segmentation makes sense of the variables in fall prevention. It is what we have attempted in defining the categories of intrinsic and extrinsic fall risks. "Multifactorial" violates these categories (even as it threads the heuristic needle and satisfies both Occam's Razor and Hickum's Dictum). In the ER it is shorthand for saying "no clearly identified single proximate cause was identified in this limited evaluation — which, by the way, is designed to diagnose and treat critical illness."

It is a shorthand that should probably be avoided. It should be replaced by a plan. Some emergency facilities are reviewing their procedures to determine if modifiable fall risks are being neglected. (They probably are.) Some are considering acute interventions by an ancillary team in the ER. At the very least, each ER should have access to a community-based falls prevention program at which they can sort out the cause of the fall by subjecting the complexity to segmentation. Most communities do not have such programs.

The same Community-based clinics should be similarly available to each person with increased risk for falling who leaves a physician's office, or is discharged from the hospital, or is the subject of an EMS (Emergency Medical Services) call, or has completed an out-patient physical therapy program.

SECTION 3
Social Darwinism

Social evolution occurs over a vastly shorter period of time than biological evolution. We evolved as an animal that ran after food and fought for territory and the right to procreate. Survival was for the fittest. Now our safety is largely assured and vast calories await us in the refrigerator. We are worse off for it. We are like a Labrador Retriever who has been given full access to the pantry. The disparity between our biology and our sociology affects the way we embrace diversity, how we structure our economy, how we wage war, how we live, and even how we die.

— Dr Arash Javanbakht, *The Conversation*[29]

When the ancestor of man was a small mammal, half-hunter and half-hunted, falling down led to eating less and being eaten more. Natural selection favored good gait because good gait granted access to resources.

Modern man still faces pressures that favor walking well, but the evolution of social supports increasingly sustain a man when walking fails. Friends help the functionally impaired to access resources, such as shelter, nutrition, healthcare, and entertainment.

But the cruel finger of natural selection, while blunted, is not gone. Some suggest that late-adult-life limitations should be viewed as beneficial from the perspectives of both biological and social evolution because they make room for the youthful to have access to resources.

In 1984, the Governor of Colorado, Richard Lamm, said, "We've got a duty to die and get out of the way with all of our machines and artificial hearts and everything else like that and let the other society, our kids, build a reasonable life."[30] He was skewered in the press for suggesting that the elderly had an obligation to use up fewer resources.

Falling is clearly not a good thing. Only a tortured logic offers that poor gait will keep a deaf man at home, safely away from where he might be run over by a bus that he cannot hear coming. But there is a limit to what friends, family, community, or government can do. At some point community resources fail, not just as resources are exhausted, but also as the tapestry of a man's biological decline overwhelms even an empathetic support network. As social support systems evolve, the point of systemic failure is simply moved further down the road.

Biologic evolution is reactive. Social systems anticipate need. They are prospective. That is why social systems evolve more rapidly than biological systems. The slower process responds to what is happening and what has happened. Long before arboreal tree mammals were part of the distant future, growing old was part of the fabric of life. The very process of aging has itself been influenced by evolution.

Said differently, biologic evolution has not been indifferent to the circumstance of the elderly, but the rules of natural selection prevailed. Social evolution has only arrived with the evolution of family, tribal, and other societal structures. And, with this has come social support networks. Some contend that such support may not be uniformly beneficial.

According to a doctrine called "Social Darwinism," as resources provided by social networks blunt the forces of natural selection, elderly man is slowly rendered less resourceful. This was a popular conservative doctrine of the late 19th century that was discredited to the extent that it supported imperialism and racism. It was embraced by Nazi Germany.

There has been a recent rebirth of interest in Social Darwinism that must be viewed with caution in a world ripe with implicit racism and laissez-faire capitalism. Notwithstanding this substantial concern, if the support extended to the elderly contributes in any way to the decline of the elderly, this should be part of the conversation. It should be discussed as a social issue right along with child abuse, access to clean water, and teen pregnancy. It is said that the best way to get out of a hole is to stop digging.

SECTION 4
Old Tools, New Tools, Theoretic Tools

Either you repeat the same conventional doctrines everybody is saying, or else you say something true, and it will sound like it is from Neptune."

— Noam Chomsky

Primary standing and walking on hind legs was a heraldic event: bipedal ambulation. Speculation about what factors favored bipedal gait has been a source of debate even before Homo erectus threw a sharp rock at Homo habilis. They were both preceded by tree-dwelling evolutionary predecessors who only used bipedal gait off and on (facultative bipedalism).

Somewhere around the time of a reptilian Hominid, a preferential stance with vertical femurs took hold. Perhaps this occurred in response to the vibrant curiosity of an enlarging brain, or to a preference to free up the revolutionary opposable thumb. Perhaps an evolution of how figs grow, moving from ground-level bushes to low-hanging fruit on trees might have stimulated standing. Locating predators over the tall grass might have allowed for motionless hiding. Clearly, being on two legs allowed more facile movement in any direction than could occur with a quadruped stance. Somehow bipedalism helped the selfish drive to access resources. Someday we may understand the factors more clearly and be enlightened.

The acquisition of this capacity in the predecessors of man was erratic, with many trial-and-error pathways and intervals of partial success. Anthropologists have traced the human bipedal lineage over 3.5 million years from the Rift Valley of Africa in several variations of hominids, along splitting pathways.[31] They have incomplete information about where and when, and similarly struggle with how. Bipedal gait is difficult. Engineers must use complex equations with non-linear differential and algebraic components applied to 4-dimensional space (whatever that is) to create an iteration of bipedal gait in modern robots.

The ability to walk on two legs was not unique to the direct ancestors of man. It is a skill that was acquired, abandoned, and then slowly learned again through countless branches on the tree of evolution over millions of years. Carnufex was a bipedal ancestor of the crocodile who ruled the dinosaurs 230 million years ago (MYA).[32] 200 MYA, Velociraptor ran down prey on its rear legs. Fossil records reveal that its front paws would not rotate downward to bear weight. He was an obligate biped.

About 150 MYA, herbivore dinosaurs, like Brachiosaurus, with huge stomachs to ferment their vegetarian diet, reverted to quadruped gait in order to carry these massive organs. Some amphibians learned to fly 120 MYA and evolved into birds. Birds are bipedal. Even the penguins who lost their ability to fly 40 MYA, remain bipedal.

Only with uninformed vanity can man view walking on two legs as something that occurred about 3.6 MYA that was a unique transition from four-legged lower mammals to man. Biblical man assumed that walking on two legs was a novelty that set him apart, and that he, not the crocodile, was created in God's image. Fully successful bipedalism still eludes us. We can do better with the application of the proper tools. Some of them are old, some are new, and some are just over the horizon.

When an adult trips on the sidewalk, there are things to do in order to reduce a recurrence. The sidewalk is repaired and the man carries himself with greater caution. If the same fall occurs with no sidewalk hazard to repair, the cause may be a deficiency in the functional capacity for not falling , and caution alone may not be the only strategy. Correction of metabolic disorders can diminish fatigue and enhance motor power. Balance issues can be addressed metabolically, by treatment of eye or ear problems, or by changes in behavior. Assistive appliances (wheelchairs, walkers, canes, grab bars, etc.) can address specific needs. Physical therapy (PT) or occupational therapy (OT) might focus on the skills of attention, power, and balance.

In elderly adults with compromised gait, conventional therapies must adapt to the restrictions of aging. For example, some can be done in a chair. Therapy can be individual or in a group setting. Tools for reacquiring the skill set of not falling have been the mainstay of conventional rehabilitation for years and have met with success.

Technology informs newer tools in physical medicine as

evidenced by the use of video and digital analysis, and applications of artificial intelligence and virtual reality. Modern surgical procedures to treat orthopedic conditions including joint replacement surgery, can reduce the consequences of pain or limited joint mobility. Because a loss of proprioception can follow these procedures, proprioceptive rehabilitation is increasingly an aspect of post-op care.[33]

There are very new tools. For example, the robots are here. Art anticipates reality. Jules Verne flew to the moon in 1865, 104 years before Neil Armstrong. In 1959 Robert Heinlein, in *Starship Troopers*, depicted robotic shells applied to the outside of men like the exoskeleton of an ant. Many recall the exo-robot worn by Sigourney Weaver in the 1986 movie *Aliens*. Now they are real.

Workplace robots can be purchased online to be worn by a worker to facilitate heavy or repetitive lifting. Paraplegics with spinal cord injuries are taking steps wearing powered exoskeletons that interface with control systems guided by nerve signals arising from the patient.[34] Soft "powered exoskeleton" underwear can supplement motor power in people with partial deficits, such as those with the power to walk but insufficient power to climb stairs.[35] Rehabilitation protocols increasingly apply exoskeleton bracing or powered exoskeleton systems to initiate early ambulation, thereby hastening the return to independent ambulation as healing occurs.

Local track systems that attach to the ceiling are available for homes. When connected to a patient harness, these permit a weak or immobile individual to be moved from toilet to sink, or lifted in or out of a bathtub (Cross-Shape, 3-Post Lift Track System, Hoyer Voyager, and others). Track systems for transfers throughout the house are available from multiple sources (T.H.E, Molift, BHM, Barrier Free, Waverley Glen, Guldman, and others).

These permanently installed tracks on the ceiling have two power sources. One lifts the patient by a cable that runs from a sling or harness worn by the patient to a housing that can glide on the track The other power source propels the housing along the track. High-tech couplings and carousels reminiscent of the track switches on a railroad allow for multiple destinations. A control box on a cable can offer independence for those able to put on their own sling. This system is currently formatted for paralyzed individuals undergoing transfers (moving or being moved from one sitting place to another). Such a system can be refined to permit fall-free assisted ambulation, perhaps with a smart phone or other voice interface to select a destination. "Alexa: Let's go to the refrigerator."

Stochastic Resonance is a tool that is based on the unlikely fact that when it comes to the brain, noise and signal within a data stream are not necessarily opposed to each other. In its most simplistic form, data arriving at the brain can reveal more than the actual content because data can be cumulative without being similar. For example, the brain reads "h7ndle" as though the 7 were an "a." The brain reads vibration (noise) from an inserted electronic sensor in a shoe as a complement to position sense data (signal) and balance is improved.[36] Applications of Stochastic Resonance will grow.

Biofeedback with NIRS (Near-Infrared Spectroscopy) will expand in the not-too-distant future. Functional NIRS is an optics technique that can measure brain or muscle activity non-invasively. This is coupled with a biofeedback paradigm in which the patient does a task and the patient or therapist watches the NIRS to see otherwise unknowable biologic response. This can create training environments for such things as relaxation training or electro-mechanical coupling of prosthetic devices.[37]

There are some tools that are purely speculative and treatments of the future are still in the realm of the theoretical.

One such possible system of care involves Planned Adaptive Gene Expression (PAGE). PAGE is designed to exploit the lessons of evolution that are retained in the DNA. The acquisition of walking without falling by an early-life toddler is echoed by the decline of gait with increased falling in late-adult life. The nervous system reverts: Once an adult, twice a child. Problems with bone and muscle, gland and organ participate in this decline, but falling in the elderly is significantly related to changes in the central nervous system — a decline in functional capacity. The nervous system components for successful gait were once "late to the party" in the 12 months post-partum toddler awaiting training and myelinization of central nervous pathways. They are once again "missing in action" in the geriatric faller. Somehow, the brain taught the toddler. PAGE suggests that in late-adult life, perhaps the maestro is capable of an encore.

A century of archeologists have tried to decipher the pathways to bipedal gait. With millions of years of evidence, accumulated bone by bone, they focused on the size and shape of the skull, the pelvis, and the extremities. Did a larger skull imply a larger brain capable of more complex motor skills and balance? Did posterior position of the hole at the base of the skull imply upright posture? Did shoulder bones with sockets directed at the horizontal suggest an animal who did not facilitate gait by hanging from higher branches? Did enlarged pelvic bones with hip sockets facing horizontally favor predominant rear extremities gait?

Speculation and dialogue generate expert opinions, and these lead to theories. Theories are then tested against fossil specimens. Those that find support are assumed to be true until replaced by better theories with better support from other bones. What was once "probably true" becomes "what we used to think." Ancient bones are relatively abundant. Soft tissues, such as make up the brain, spinal cord, and muscle, are not part of the fossil record.

The brain is an organ with the consistency of week-old tapioca, barely able to support itself. It works with rapidly shifting electrical and chemical interactions. Change is what it does. The bones do a few things, and the brain does many. This is referred to as having different "degrees of freedom." The more degrees of freedom that exist the more trials of different pathways and mechanisms can occur. The opportunity for evolutionary change is greater in the more complex organ. While motor skill and general function evolve in harmony with the bones of the skeleton, the ability to walk on two legs is more clearly the consequence of evolution of the brain than evolution of the leg.

Much of what we know about brain evolution is informed speculation. Actual data from the study of muscle, nerve, and brain tissue from ancestral mammals is scant. A window through which to view the evolution of the pathway to bipedal gait is missing.

When the skills needed to avoid falling decline in disease or in late adulthood, knowledge of how man initially acquired bipedal gait could be useful. The pathway to acquisition could offer a manual on how to reacquire this eroded functional capacity, if only there were a window into this knowledge. Man embodies the sum of millions of years of evolution. Toddlers live it. They will be our window.

Long before becoming a toddler, the embryonic states of the human animal retraces evolutionary history: ontogeny recapitulates phylogeny. Embryos retrace the path of all evolution in a pattern called embryological parallelism.

Mammalian biology begins its human journey on this planet as a fertilized egg, a single cell amoeba-like organism that burrows into the obliging wall of the uterus. Supported there, cellular division begins under the orderly instructions of DNA. First it is a hydra-like organism that appears ancestral to a squid. This soon develops fish-like gills, and later amphibian-like appendages, before it shoulders a mammalian "evolve." That's a lot of change for a little kid, and it doesn't stop.

Infants are thrust into a non-aquatic, air-breathing world with gravity and a mandate to seek nutrition. They crawl, quadruped-style. Then, driven by some primordial need they stand and, after a bit of bouncing in place, they walk, biped. They are retracing the trail of man, recapitulating that phylogeny thing.

They toddle with arms outstretched like someone accustomed to grabbing branches. They fall. Injuries are limited by short stature and the caution of others. They get up again, better informed about the indignities of falling. A slowly maturing brain coordinates strategies to do better next time. Before long next time is running on a playground, then in a gymnasium, and then in an Olympic stadium, or perhaps simply performing activities of daily living.

And they still may fall, but time has wrought two guardians: skill and anticipation. Skill is the intrinsic ability to halt a near fall. Anticipation is knowledge of a risk or hazard, with attention to the present in the service of the future. Then, over the decades, skill and anticipation erode. Again, as Shakespeare said, "Once an adult and twice a child." Aging, tall, and bipedal, with the journey of a lifetime aching in joints, falling in the elderly increasingly seems inevitable.

The DNA that orchestrated the initial acquisition of gait at age 14 months is still there. Theoretically, if we are clever enough we should be able turn it on, like we do with the alpha-neuron gene with exercise. Cancer doctors are learning how to use drugs to turn on genes which increase the sensitivity of a tumor cell to chemotherapy. Neurology does yet have this, but perhaps we can learn how to turn on the genes needed to reacquire lost gait by studying the initial acquisition of gait by toddlers.

Observation is a semi-quantitative and non-invasive tool. Watch toddlers in the bus terminal or toy store. Not all kids are the same. You might see anything from slow, flat-footed prudency, to a ballistic Cotton-Eyed Joe. But most approach gait in a fairly uniform fashion, with a high-contact short stride, wide base, elbows back with abbreviated arm swing and palms facing forward. The cadence is semi-rapid and semi-rhythmic. Feet are flat with most of the time in the gait cycle spent with both feet contacting the floor. They fall, land on their bum, roll, move back to standing, and shortly fall on their bum again.

Over several months, falling forward becomes a more common risk. Most kids will land on their chin and some will do so more than once before the negative feedback and improving skill conspire to make them land on their hands and knees. Skills improve with time. Walking soon gives way to walking fast and this soon gives way to running.

Falls continue to occur, but less often. They persist with a biologic certitude, a success bias, that neglects past failures and embraces each new triumph. They are expressing lessons learned by ancestral primates who moved down to the floor of the forest and ventured across the savannahs, dragging their forelimbs on front-facing knuckles until they learned otherwise. By age 3-6 years you can hardly knock kids over.

Witnessing a baby creep, then crawl, then toddle and walk are joyous and heartwarming. Muscle power and bone strength, heart and lung capacity, brain function — all are necessary, none are sufficient . The brain appears to be the rate-limiting step.

In infancy, the rate at which gait is acquired is dictated by brain maturation. The central nervous system is rightly viewed as "late to the party." Humans are born with a brain half-baked. The laying down of insulation, myelination, continues long after birth, and is not fully finished for decades. As pathways in the brain and spinal cord myelinate, they conduct electrical impulses more rapidly, moving information from one area to many areas.

Complex behavior, like walking and not falling, requires the rapid distribution of vast amounts of information. Nonetheless, gait actually comes fairly early. The skill set for Not Falling is being acquired at the time that the concepts of yes and no are still a rudimentary puzzle. Walking becomes an established skill at about the same time the child has acquired about 100 words. The young master of syntax walks over and says "Me ran fast. Me go ride the Roundi-Go?"

Planned Adaptive Gene Expression, PAGE, aspires to place the elderly person who has experienced recurrent falls in a circumstance that emulates or recaps their time as a toddler. The expectation is that PAGE training will cause a regression that activates genes that have been silent, and that the expression of these genes will be adaptive to the reacquisition of gait. The elementary PAGE plan for falls prevention in a late-aged adult, a physical medicine approach with a four-step program, might look like this: It begins with an odd proposition that "arms are for walking."

PAGE Plan

STEP 1: ARMS ARE FOR WALKING

The subject is instructed to keep his or her elbows back with arms gently flexed at the elbow and with hands pronated throughout all phases of the gait cycle. Pay attention to arm swing, heel strike, and stride line.

Walking follows the "gait cycle," the predictable arm and leg swings and weight transfers. The gait cycle begins from a stance position. Then, during brief full weight bearing on the right foot. the left leg strides forward (left leg swing phase). With the left foot heel strike, weight begins to distribute bilaterally, and as the left foot rolls from heel toward toe (follows a stride line), brief full weight bearing on the left foot permits the right leg swing phase, and so on.

The swing phase is not launched randomly. The most effective trajectory is aimed forward, directly down what is called the "line of gait." Rotational hip girdle energy is applied to overcome the inertia of the dangling leg to get it to move forward, and this energy tends to rotate the hip girdle backwards, in a direction that would send the left leg toward the left (or the right leg toward the right), well off the line of gait.

But, at the same time as the left leg swings forward, the left arm swings toward the rear. The arm momentum places rotational force on the hip girdle equal to and in the reverse direction from the forces being applied at the same moment by the hip girdle to initiate the left leg swing phase. Therefore, the left leg is launched correctly down the line of gait because of the left arm rearward swing. As the gait cycle proceeds, the right leg is launched straight down the line of gait because of right arm rearward swing. Arms are for walking.

All of this works best when mechanoreceptors in the skin, muscles, tendons, and joint inform the central nervous system where things are and how positions are changing. The arm of an adult has evolved for fine motor skills so it is better at accumulating and transmitting information than the leg. Arm mechanoreceptors are more sensitive than those in leg joints and muscles.

This differential of arms over legs is especially true in late adult life. When the elderly have age-related failure of mechanoreceptors and slowed data transmission in nerves, the further the data is from the central nervous system the worse the effects of this failure. Arms are much shorter than legs, and offer relatively expedited access to central processing centers. From a proprioceptive perspective, arms are for walking.

An indifferent hanging arm requires less force to swing backwards than one flexed at the elbow. Therefore, a flexed left arm applies greater force at the left hip than an extended arm, causing more forceful guidance to the left leg to stride forward in the swing phase without leaving the line of gait. Just as they were for the toddler, with arms flexed, elbows back and exaggerated arm swing, arms are for walking.

And pronated hands (turned so that the palm is facing downward or forward)? Clinicians have recognized a process called "anterior carrying angle of the arms" in many neurodegenerative disease. This is a preferential posture when gait declines in which the palm of the hand is carried facing the front of the hip rather than the usual adult posture in which the palm of the hand faces the side of the hip. The hands and forearms have instinctively pronated. Forearm pronation with the elbow flexed forces the elbow away from the body. This adds further rotational force to the hip as the arm swings to the rear, and this enhances control of the ipsilateral leg swing phase, as previously described. Arms are for walking.

STEP 2: GAIT'S GOT RHYTHM

The subject begins with comfortably short strides with a mildly widened base. As progress is identified, increase the frequency or cadence to approximately two per second with a short stride before any attempt to increase the stride length. Walk from one large object of support to another. Hand, arm, and elbow postures are as noted in Step 1.

This is what you will see toddlers do when you watch them acquire gait. The rapid stride cadence may be a recapitulation of the pervasive maternal heartbeat that filled their world for nine months. Recent literature instructs first responders to perform cardiac compressions at the cadence of the 1977 Bee Gees song "Stayin' Alive." Tribal music, klezmer, bhangra and hip hop/rap, each offer a possible rhythm for PAGE. PAGE is best done to the right music if the patient is receptive.

STEP 3: LEARNING IS RISKY BUSINESS

The subject increases his or her stride length incrementally. This may require harness support to permit sufficient cadence and repetitions. Instruct in falls risk. Hand, arm, and elbow posture are as noted in Step 1.

Toddlers lengthen their stride length at about the time they begin to run. This process often involves a transition from falling on the bum to falling on the face, and is a phase that elderly people must be aware of and work to avoid as much as possible.

STEP 4: ALL'S WELL THAT FALLS WELL

The subject will receive instructions concerning how to fall without injury, and how to get up with or without assistance.

Toddlers are persistent in their pursuit of success. They fall throughout their youth and with practice they learn to do it well.

They are resilient. The elderly, after a life of learning by avoiding failure, approach falling differently. Falling has been so avoided that there is hardly any retained skill-set for how to do it well. Falling well is critical to being able to persist. Whether taught by conventional physical therapy methods or by the martial arts falling techniques (Ukemi), falling properly can reduce the harm of falls even in those with doubtful resilience.[38]

When physical medicine becomes more vain and recognizes that physical therapy is genetic manipulation, it will more fully leverage the lessons of evolution.

Section 5
A Proprioceptive Appliance

Research by Paul Bach-y-Rita 60 years ago on plasticity (adaptability) of the brain described a man with no vision who was being trained to "see" the room via a TV camera.[39] The camera activated an array of vibrating plates on a chair. These plates rested against the man's back. Each active pixel on the TV was represented by a small plate. For example, the letter T, placed in front of the camera, activated a T-shaped cluster of vibrating plates on his back. The man did not appear to be making much real progress in learning to discern objects. One day an errant beach ball came flying at the camera, and the man reflexively recoiled. Tactile skin information had been processed by his brain and triggered a rapid instinctive reflex as though he had seen it. The event that day was the proprioceptive equivalent of reading Braille.

Sensory function keeps track of spatial relationships. Vision can keep track of the spatial relationships of things which emit or reflect light. The inner ear can keep track of spatial relationships defined by lateral acceleration of the head, or by hearing the time disparity between the arrival of acoustic information at each cochlea.

Tactile skin sensation can keep track of spatial relationships that touch, press, or stretch the surface of the body. Mechanoreceptors in skin, muscles, tendons and joints can keep track of spatial relationships that stretch or compress them. The sensory capacity called proprioception combines any of the sources of measurement that are available into a coherent data stream. In a dark room it preferentially will stream mechanoreceptor data. When the legs are numb, data can be redirected through the arm or trunk. By these measures, proprioception has innate plasticity. This plasticity raises the likelihood that retraining is a reasonable goal.

The white cane used by a blind man is not anticipated to carry weight. It is to substitute tactile information for the absent visual information. This reduces falls by allowing the man to identify extrinsic hazards. Additionally, the vibration and displacement of the white cane contribute to a proprioceptive stream of information that reduces falls by supporting the intrinsic capacity for not falling. Some of this may involve stochastic resonance, which was reviewed in Chapter 3, section 4.

The purpose of a conventional cane is to carry some weight. The amount is determined by the nature of the gait disorder and can vary between circumstances. A conventional cane is not meant to avoid extrinsic hazards like the white cane of the blind man. It may contribute to the proprioceptive stream of information, but it is not especially well designed to do so because this role is blunted by weight-bearing. It does not support the intrinsic capacity for not falling as well as a cane of alternate design and purpose.

In a late-age adult the stream of proprioceptive information declines. A large part of this decline reflects lost data from the legs. Mechanoreceptors age in poorly defined ways, and are probably subject to specific disease states that are not yet defined. They begin to send imprecise data. The transmission of this data through aging nerves is slowed and this especially impacts data flowing in the physically long nerves in the legs.

Unreliable or incomplete "elderly "data also flows from the eyes and the ears. This diminished proprioceptive stream arrives at brain and spinal centers themselves slowed by aging. This conspiracy reduces the intrinsic capacity for not falling. Increasing the accuracy and the amount of proprioceptive data, and the speed with which it is transmitted to the brain and spinal cord will logically stabilize or reverse this process.

The design of canes and walking sticks has been largely unchanged for centuries and apart from their grip, they are straight. Even in those with decorative curves, the tip contacts the floor directly below, or nearly directly below, the grip. This is helpful for weight bearing. A cane offers a third point of contact with the ground, which helps create a stable base. The cane provides the hand and arm with some limited data about where the ground is. This data flows through relatively efficient pathways to the brain and spinal cord. A differently designed assistive device can offer an increase in stability of the base and improve upon the accuracy and amount of proprioceptive data being sent.

A properly curved cane, with a grip that assures that the convexity of the curve faces forward, will cause the tip of the cane to contact the floor ahead of the grip, that is, several inches further down the line of gait. This is called forward placement. The average conventional cane encounters the floor at a point approximately parallel to the toe of the opposite foot during the forward stride portion of the gait cycle. That is, with the cane held in the right hand, the left leg strides forward with a completed heel-strike, but the right leg has not yet begun to stride forward. Then, the cane tip, carried forward by the right arm swing, encounters the floor about as far down the line of gait as the toe of the left shoe.

Under the same circumstance, the tip of the curved cane encounters the floor as much as 12 inches forward of the toe of the left shoe. The location of the tip is not well-suited to weight bearing, but it offers two benefits. The forward placement creates a third point of contact with the ground that forms a broader tripod than that associated with the tip location of a conventional cane. This creates a more stable base.

Secondly, it acquires proprioceptive data, not unlike that acquired by a blind man's white cane. Like the conventional cane, the curved cane gains access to the brain via the efficient pathways of the arm. The alternate design and purpose of a proprioceptive appliance will be useful for fall prevention in disorders of balance, that is, conditions in which the deficit is predominantly proprioceptive.

SECTION 6
Behavioral Obstacles? Attitude This!

If everybody was satisfied with himself there would be no heroes.

—Samuel Clemens, Mark Twain's Autobiography

In 1986 Ronald Reagan humorously described the nine most terrifying words on earth as: "I'm from the government and I'm here to help you." The recent track record of the government in extending "help" to the elderly is terrifying in the extent to which it is complicated. United States legislative undertakings read like the ancestral lineage of the Old Testament. Read on.

The Older Americans Act of 1965 (OAA) established a national network of federal, state, and local agencies to plan for and provide services to help older adults live independently in their homes and communities. This act gave rise to an interconnected structure of agencies known as the "Aging Network," run by the Administration on Aging. The Aging Network begat 56 state agencies on aging, more than 260 Title VI Native American aging programs and 622 Area Agencies on Aging (AAA). These coordinate with and are supported by tens of thousands of academic and professional organizations, service providers, and volunteers.

The 622 Area Agencies on Aging form the National Association of Area Agencies on Aging (N4A) to help Washington set priorities, and build the capacity of the member Area Agencies on Aging to a create "a society that values and supports people as they age." Each Area Agency on Aging (AAA) serves a city or region and provides a variable suite of services. These include nutrition assistance, respite care for caregivers, long term care ombudsmen, transportation, health and welfare information, and referrals. The Area Agency on Aging begat The National Resource Center for Engaging Older Adults (engAGED).

The government is not alone. National and regional organizations are also working to help the aged. The National Council on Aging (NCOA), is a nonprofit organization started 69 years ago that "brings together nonprofit organizations, businesses, and government to develop creative solutions that improve the lives of older adults." Their budget is knit together from federal, state, local and charitable sources. In 2017 the direct NCOA budget exceeded $50 million dollars, and they connected individuals with over $1 billion in resources. More than 600,000 elderly adults participated in their disease management or falls prevention workshops. The NCOA supports community centers and programs for the elderly. It establishes "best practices" for assisting the aged, and offers online tools and tips to stay healthy and economically secure. It provides the latest in aging policy to advocate for the elderly and teaches them how to speak up for seniors in need. The NCOA is the parent organization of the National Institute of Senior Centers (NISC). This organization supports a national network of over 2,000 senior center professionals "dedicated to helping older adults remain active, engaged, and independent in their communities."

Each year falls result in an increasing number of emergency room visits, hospitalizations, and deaths. The government is helping. Not-for-profit organizations and agencies are helping. Non-Government Organizations from churches to AARP to the American Association of Occupational Therapy are helping. Charities and volunteers are helping. The effort is large, focused, and yet insufficient.

Here is the problem. In 2017, the United States Department of Housing and Urban Development (HUD) published *Overcoming Obstacles to Policies for Preventing Falls by the Elderly,*[40] a stunningly thorough analysis of the obstacles encountered by communities in developing and implementing policies and programs to prevent falls in late-age adults. Federal, state, and local policies were painstakingly reviewed by a panel of experts from government and academic centers. Three primary obstacles were identified. The first was a legislative obstacle: the lack of long-term coordinated funding.

The second was a scientific obstacle: the lack of uniformity in research methodology. The third obstacle to the successful implementation of falls prevention programs was the inability to recruit and engage seniors in fall prevention programs.

Each of these obstacles requires a tactical adjustment. Improved tactics for the coordinated funding obstacle will be handled by bureaucrats and research obstacles will be handled by academics. New tactics to overcome the behavioral obstacle of deficient participation will need to arise from thinking outside of the bureaucratic box.

The people to whom the help is offered, at whom the legislation is aimed, for whom the research is done, are the very people among whom participation lags. The goal is to reduce falls. The strategy is to increase participation. An adjustment in tactics is needed for the strategy to succeed.

As noted in earlier chapters, late-aged adults have risk factors for falling might one day be classified as extrinsic factors, socio-demographic factors, intrinsic factors, and behavioral factors. Interestingly, these are also the risk factors for failure to participate. The tactics to gain participation in fall prevention programs have focused on these four areas in the past. These areas need new tactical approaches.

Extrinsic factors that affect participation in fall prevention programs are already being addressed. Tactics to overcome them are increasingly imaginative and helpful.

For example, in rural communities social service sites may be few and far between. Local church and school-based programs help, and travel-assistance programs have success. Sociodemographic tactics can be applied, including subsidizing the cost of the program or the expense of missing work. Exercise friendly multigenerational parks are on the drawing boards. Cultural restrictions that, for example, might discourage women from comfortably participating in exercise with men, are helped with single-sex group exercise or private therapy. Immigrant populations are contacted within their individual communities and in their own language.

Intrinsic reasons for failure to participate in falls prevention programs also receive attention. Transportation assistance or home programs are made available for those too impaired to travel due to things like gait disorders, frailty, or vision loss. Exercise groups include standing and seated exercise concurrently. Services include home assessment tours to identify hazards for falling in those too infirm or socially isolated to perform the assessment independently.

The government and the community have tactics to address behavioral obstacles. Cities sponsor regional information campaigns and outreach programs from community centers. Most states sponsor a Falls Prevention Day with billboards on highways and banners on buses. Adult Living Facilities present fall prevention programs as a social activity. Nearly all programs encourage family participation, tracking of progress, and efforts to be culturally sensitive. Exercise leaders are taught to be sensitive to individual capacities and to recognize that each person has a need to be encouraged and a need for positive reinforcement.

These tactics work. Oregon celebrates Falls Prevention Day. Hawaii celebrates Falls Prevention Week, and fully funds seven regional centers that provide free Tai Chi (a group exercise program with proven success in fall prevention). Hawaii has far fewer elderly falls per capita than Oregon.

Most of these tactics were already in place when the HUD 2017 study was done. Perhaps this simply reflects that change can be slow even in the face of good tactics. Universal suffrage became the law of the land in 1921, but 1980 was the first year that woman voted at the same rate as men. It might also be evidence of a tactical deficiency. It would be worth considering if something is being missed in the tactics used to gain participation of late-age adults in falls prevention programs.

Behaviors that are familiar are embraced, especially by the elderly. New and unfamiliar things are slow to take root. Participation in community-based group exercise, or in a social support network , or a home assessment tour to identify fall hazards come under the heading of "new things."

Neurologists observe that as a person ages they often "become themselves, but more so." A curt young man becomes a crotchety old guy. An egotistical middle-aged woman becomes a dowager queen. Said differently, in the later years of life attitudes and styles stop being filtered. They assert command. John Maxwell says, in *Attitude 101: What Every Leader Needs to Know*,[41] "attitude is never content until it is expressed. It is the librarian of the past...the speaker of the present...the prophet of the future."

It is worth recalling the definition of attitude: "a settled way of thinking or feeling about someone or something that is reflected in a person's behavior." A partial list of attitudes that might reduce participation in a fall prevention program includes vain, shy, angry, stubborn, nihilistic, indifferent, and hopeless. Each arises from a place that the individual has grown to view as intensely personal and reasonable — their comfort zone.

Late-age adults embrace their attitudes as insurmountable This is unfortunate since attitudes that reduce participation increase falling, and falling is unsatisfactory. There is a lesson to be learned about attitudes and behaviors in later adult life, and this lesson leads to a tactic.

In the first years of a medical practice, a young physician will often be surprised by the inability of an otherwise intact patient to provide a coherent rendition of their symptoms, "a good history." Medical thinking is different than regular thinking. Focus is ajar. For a patient, the intensity and urgency of "it" are the focus, often to the relative exclusion of saying what "it" is.

Words offer challenges. Numbness and weakness fully overlap in the mind of a patient. Dizziness can mean almost anything. It takes three or four years of medical practice to learn how to extract a coherent history. It takes 20 years to realize that patients conceal information without being conscious of the intent to do so; they conceal from the doctor that which they conceal from themselves. A seasoned doctor begins to hear more than he is being told when he acknowledges his patient's vulnerability: They will misrepresent or neglect those things that they find to be unsatisfactory.

Morris came to see me four years after a "stupid injury." In the course of a pleasant afternoon drinking beer with old friends, this group of 50-year-old men began an ill-advised game of touch football. It ended in his left shoulder being dislocated. When he left the ER that day with persistent pain and arm weakness, Morris felt more like he had failed an IQ test than some physical challenge. When the process took nearly a year to resolve he felt "disappointed and stupid."

When he came to see me four years later, it was to get help for mild persistent arm pain and a vexing unrelenting sensation that he called "fatigue." Upon examination, his shoulder demonstrated evidence of mild weakness, numbness, and muscle atrophy which corresponded to the malfunction of a specific nerve that was, regrettably, damaged at the time of his shoulder injury.

He had been advised that healing had occurred, that intervention was not necessary, and that further recovery was unlikely. He knew all that. "But what about the damned fatigue?"

This sensation he called fatigue was thoroughly unacceptable.

Using lessons taught to me by patients over the years, we soon agreed that his word "fatigue" was imprecise, and placed an unnecessary burden on clarity. It was not the bone-weary fatigue of lifting hundred-pound sacks of corn. Fatigue was the best word he could find. What he meant was that the persistent mild weakness and numbness felt abnormal and "unsatisfactory." Soon he realized that while "fatigue" was a sign of something that might demand attention, "unsatisfactory" was a perspective that he might simply choose to ignore. And that is what he did. And ten years later he is not vexed, and he participates in many activities. Abnormal is unsatisfactory. Deal with it and move on.

Aging is unsatisfactory in the sort of comparative way that riding a bike with flat tires is unsatisfactory. Fully-pumped tires flatten the ruts in the road. The mind is free to smell the roses along the trail. With flat tires the ruts prevail. Discomfort and the risk of toppling lurk around every bend. Risk siphons away attention and threatens each chance to smell the roses, each chance for joy. A normal adult (full tires), compares himself to an aged adult (flat tires). Unsatisfactory!

In Caligula, Albert Camus writes: "To lose one's life is no great matter; when the time comes I'll have the courage to lose mine. But what's intolerable is to see one's life being drained of meaning." A loss of purpose and functional capacity sucks away meaning. Aging often does this.

Even those advanced-age adults with a positive attitude, who continue take on new invigorating burdens, often do so with a quiet sense that things may be unsatisfactory. They may be role models to their peers, but they remain unwittingly vulnerable. When Morris grew to recognized this vulnerability, he participated. He became a better role model.

Here is another instructive case: "Ducks! Do they think that I'm an idiot? They want to take me over to the pond to look at the ducks and they call that a tour?"

Bertha is an uncommonly bright woman of 95 years. She has spent much of the last 25 years reading novels and writing two of her own. Three years ago she was "forced" out of "her beloved condominium" and into an apartment in a medium-sized adult living facility. She is not unfamiliar with a lingering dislike for the management. Her disdain for the dining room staff and for the quality of the food is something she shares with many of her neighbors. In reality, the food, the management, and the staff are satisfactory. Her complaining about it is a proxy for her dissatisfaction with growing old and dependent, and for being coerced out of "her beloved condominium." (All of which she will occasionally briefly endorse as true.)

Fellow residents who do not recall her name refer to her as "the lady who always smiles." She is often a calm thoughtful advocate for all of them, but this duck business was a step too far. Her disdain found voice early and often. It seemed indifferent to who she is — to deny who she had once been. This struck too close to home. She was enraged.

After some brief investigation, it became evident that the "duck tour" notice was for an energetic and appealing adventure on a "duck boat", an amphibious vehicle that would load up tourists on dry land and then drive into the watery Everglades to see the plants, the wading birds, and the alligators. When this was pointed out to Bertha, she never mentioned it again. Even in her relative hardiness she is clearly vulnerable to her harshest critic — herself. She makes behavioral decisions based on her attitude. And despite a full life with family and career, with aging her attitude mirrors "unsatisfactory."

Here then is an "outside of the box" tactical option, offered in the hope that attitude in the aged does not actually have insurmountable momentum. Programs for fall prevention have learned many helpful tactics for recruiting and retaining participants, and they must continue to apply these, to cast themselves as convenient and helpful and fun and free and culturally appropriate. But, they also need to "get real" and acknowledge something: life for many late-aged adults has become unsatisfactory. War is hell. Black is beautiful. The emperor is naked — and old age is unsatisfactory.

When the opportunity to participate in a new falls prevention program presents itself we should lead them to say: "My dear friend, as unsatisfactory as old age may appear to be, it is not simply a condition. It is a perspective, and the option to change is mine. Choice is mine. Unsatisfactory is a sauce in which my attitudes have marinated. But I have unfinished business. I will not go gentle into that good night. This is an opportunity to change my behavior."

Leading a person with risk for falling to this conclusion can be left to community outreach, but it is often a role for the caregiver. A positive role can be played by "mini-caregivers," such as nieces, nephews, neighbors and friends who stay in contact and realize that their love and attention has a robust impact on the attitudes of the elderly. Attitude this: *Participate!*

If we address this, will all the other tactics we have learned to apply be more effective? With this simple truth of perspective and attitude acknowledged, will the elderly be more likely to embrace an opportunity for fewer falls and less pain? Of course! Change the tactics. Change the attitudes. Change the behaviors. Change the future.

NOTES

[25] S. Daniele Physical Exercise as an Epigenetic Modulator: Eustress, "The 'Positive Stress' as an Effector of Gene Expression," *Journal of Strength and Conditioning Research*, 26(12):3469–3472, December 2012 DOI: 10.1519/ JSC.0b013e31825bb594.

[26] Balance and Fall Prevention Training for the Active Adult https://www.bosu.com/blog/cat/active-aging/.

[27] Do-yeon Kim, MPT, PT1 and Chae-gil Lim, PhD, PT2, "Effects of Pedalo® training on balance and fall risk in stroke patients," *Journal of Physical Therapy Science*,. 2017 Jul; 29(7): 1159–1162 Published online 2017 Jul 15. doi: 10.1589/jpts.29.1159.

[28] Ruopeng Sun and Jacob Sosnoff, "Novel sensing technology in fall risk assessment in older adults: a systematic review," BMC Geriatrics. 2018; 18: 14. Published online 2018 Jan 16. doi: 10.1186/s12877-018-0706-6   PMID: 29338695.

[29] Arash Javanbakht, The Conversation: To live your best life, live the life you evolved for,. (https://www.cnn.com/2019/02/04/health/life-you-evolved-for-partner/index.html), Updated 2:50 AM ET, Tue February 5, 2019.

[30] *New York Times*, March 29, 1984 Gov, Lamm asserts "Elderly, if very ill, have "duty to die."

[31] Mark A Maslina, Chris M Brierley, Alic M Milnara, "East African climate pulses and early human evolution," *Quaternary Science Reviews,* Volume 101, 1 October 2014, Pages 1-17.

[32] Crocodile Ancestor Was Top Predator Before Dinosaurs Roamed North America, https://news.ncsu.edu/2015/03/zanno-carnufex/   accessed 8/24/2019.

[33] Tolga Saka, "Principles of postoperative anterior cruciate ligament rehabilitation," *World Journal of Orthopedics*, 2014 Sep 18; 5(4): 450–459.

[34] Ashraf S Gorgey, "Robotic exoskeletons: The current pros and cons," *World Journal of Orthopedics*, 2018 Sep 18; 9(9): 112–119. Published online 2018 Sep 18. doi: 10.5312/wjo.v9.i9.112

[35] Soft Exosuits, https://biodesign.seas.harvard.edu/soft-exosuits accessed 8/24/2019,

[36] Oliver White, Jan Babie, Carlos Trenado Leif Johannsen Nandu Goswani, "The Promise of Stochastic Resonance in Falls Prevention," *Frontiers in Physiology*, 28 January 2019 | https://doi.org/10.3389/fphys.2018.01865.

[37] Masahito Mihari and Ichiro Miyail, "Review of functional near-infrared spectroscopy in neurorehabilitation," *Neurophotonics,* 2016 Jul; 3(3): 031414. Published online 2016 Jul 12. doi: 0.1117/1.NPh.3.3.0314141.

[38] Can martial arts falling techniques prevent injuries? https://injuryprevention.bmj.com/content/9/3/284.1.full accessed 6/24/2019.

[39] Paul Bach-y-Rita, Frank Saunders, Benjamin White, "Vision Substitution by Tactile Image Projection," *Nature*, volume 221, pages963–964 (1969).

[40] Overcoming Obstacles to Effective Senior Falls Prevention and Coordinated Care, https://www.hud.gov/sites/documents/SENIORFALLS_TOOLKIT.PDF accessed 7/16/2019.

[41] John C Maxwell, *Leadership*, Harper Collins, 1/1/2003, 22.

EPILOGUE

My grandmother started walking five miles a day when she was sixty. She's ninety-seven now, and we don't know where the hell she is.

— Ellen DeGeneres[42]

At some point, after exploring the extrinsic and the intrinsic, applications and speculations, the time comes to be concise: It takes individual effort not to fall and it takes a strategy. The strategy laid out in this book is at a somewhat granular level. Review the data, be informed, gain insight, and become wise.

The approach might not suit everyone. For those in search of a quicker fix, ask your doctor for a fall risk assessment, engage in regular exercise, and perform an assessment of your home to make changes to reduce risks.[43] Do something. Even an ostrich does not actually bury its head in the sand. Yogi Berra, baseball great and hero of my youth famously instructed us all: "when you come to a fork in the road, take it."

---

[42] Ellen DeGeneres, https://wealthygorilla.com/40-wonderful-ellen-degeneres-quotes/ accessed 8/25/2019.

[43] Catch Yourself: Simple Steps to Prevent Falls, http://www.stopfalls.org/resources/downloadables/catch_yourself.pdf.

APPENDIX
INTERNET RESOURCES

Martin Menkin, MD, Intrinsic and Extrinsic Factors in Fall Prevention

https://www.notfalling.net/

The University of Southern California Leonard Davis School of Gerontology

Falls Prevention Center of Excellence (stopfalls.org)

Home Modification Resource Inventories
http://stopfalls.org/resources/home-modification-tools-programs-and-funding-landingpage/

National Council on Aging (ncoa.org)

Fall Prevention
https://www.ncoa.org/healthy-aging/falls-prevention/

Falls Free Initiative. National Falls Prevention Action Plan 2015
https://www.ncoa.org/healthy-aging/falls-prevention/falls-free-initiative/

National Association of Area Agencies on Aging (n4a.org)

Preventing Falls at Home
https://www.n4a.org/files/PreventingFalls.pdf

The National Aging in Place Council (NAICP)

http://www.ageinplace.org/

National Institutes of Health, National Institute on Aging (nih.nia.gov)

Falls and Fall Prevention
https://www.nia.nih.gov/health/topics/falls-and-falls-prevention

Center for Disease Control (cdc.gov)

Take a Stand on Falls
https://www.cdc.gov/features/older-adult-falls

Check for Safety. A Home Fall Prevention Checklist
https://www.cdc.gov/HomeandRecreationalSafety/pubs/English/booklet_Eng_desktop-a.pdf

Housing and Urban Development (hud.gov)

Home Modification Guide
https://www.hud.gov/sites/documents/HOME_MOD_GUIDE.PDF

Overcoming Obstacles to Effective Senior Falls Prevention and Coordinated Care
https://www.hud.gov/sites/documents/SENIORFALLS_TOOLKIT.PDF

Housing for Seniors: Challenges and Solutions
https://www.hud.gov/sites/documents/SENIORFALLS_TOOLKIT.PDF

STEADI. Stop Elderly Accidents Deaths and Injury
https//www.hud.gov/sites/documents/SENIORFALLS_TOOLKIT.PDF

American Occupational Therapy Association, Inc (aota.org.)

Falls Prevention
https://www.aota.org/falls

American Physical Therapy Association (apta.org)

Balance and Falls
http://www.apta.org/BalanceFalls/

AARP (aarp.org)

Caregiving Checklist: Preventing Falls
https://assets.aarp.org/external_sites/caregiving/checklists/checklist_preventFalls.html

Caregiving Checklist: Home Safety
https://assets.aarp.org/external_sites/caregiving/checklists/checklist_homeSafety.htm

www.ingramcontent.com/pod-product-compliance
Lightning Source LLC
Chambersburg PA
CBHW050736030426
42336CB00012B/1597